AME 科研时间系列医学图书 1B066

病例报告撰写规范 CARE 解读

主　编：张开平

副主编：韩金鸣　戴晨阳　贾林沛　姜　龙　花苏榕

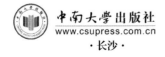
中南大学出版社
www.csupress.com.cn
·长沙·

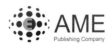
AME
Publishing Company

图书在版编目（CIP）数据

病例报告撰写规范CARE解读/张开平主编．—长沙：中南大学出版社，2022.10

ISBN 978 - 7 - 5487 - 5021 - 5

Ⅰ．①病…　Ⅱ．①张…　Ⅲ．①病案—书写规则　Ⅳ．①R197.323

中国版本图书馆CIP数据核字(2022)第135907号

AME 科研时间系列医学图书 1B066

病例报告撰写规范 CARE 解读

BINGLIBAOGAO ZHUANXIEGUIFAN CARE JIEDU

主　编：张开平

□出 版 人	吴湘华
□丛书策划	汪道远　陈海波
□项目编辑	陈海波　廖莉莉
□责任编辑	陈海波　彭敏宁　李沛宇　黄冰滢
□责任印制	唐　曦　潘飘飘
□版式设计	朱三萍　林子钰
□出版发行	中南大学出版社

社址：长沙市麓山南路　　　　　　邮编：410083

发行科电话：0731-88876770　　　传真：0731-88710482

□策 划 方　AME Publishing Company

地址：香港沙田石门京瑞广场一期，16 楼 C

网址：www.amegroups.com

□印　　装　天意有福科技股份有限公司

□开　　本　710×1000　1/16　□印张 5.75　□字数 109 千字　□插页

□版　　次　2022 年 10 月第 1 版　□2022 年 10 月第 1 次印刷

□书　　号　ISBN 978 - 7 - 5487 - 5021 - 5

□定　　价　185.00 元

编者风采

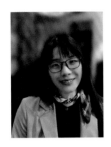

主编：张开平

AME出版社

PhD，MPH，药理学博士，公共卫生学硕士，主要负责AME出版社旗下多本SCI等英文期刊医学评论稿件的邀约及自由投稿的编辑部内审，包括对稿件质量和报告质量的审查。《手术技术报告指南》（*Surgical techniqUe rePorting chEcklist and standaRds*，*SUPER*）的主要制定人之一，以第一/通讯作者发表英文学术论文近20篇。主译《生物医学研究报告指南：用户手册》，参编《观察性研究论文撰写规范STROBE解读》。

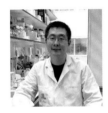

副主编：韩金鸣

首都医科大学宣武医院神经内科

瑞典卡罗林斯卡医学院临床神经科学系博士，现首都医科大学宣武医院神经内科博士后，欧洲免疫学会和国际免疫学会会员，中国神经科学学会神经免疫学分会会员，主要从事神经免疫性疾病基础研究和临床工作。目前已发表SCI文章40余篇，被引用600余次，担任50余本SCI期刊独立审稿人，如*Frontiers in immunology*、*Molecular Neurobiology*、*Oxidative Medicine and Cellular Longevity*、*Neurology and Therapy*、*Translational Neurodegeneration*，累计审稿200余次。目前担任*BMC Neurology*和*Frontiers in Bioscience-Landmark*期刊编委，*Annals of Translational Medicine*、*Traditional Medicine Research*和《中华生物医学工程杂志》中青年编委，*Frontiers in Neurology*和*Disease Markers*客座编辑。参与科技部国家重点研发计划1项，参与国家自然科学基金面上项目1项，获得吉林省科技进步二等奖1项。

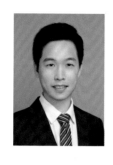

副主编：戴晨阳

同济大学附属上海市肺科医院胸外科

医学博士，同济大学附属上海市肺科医院胸外科主治医师，同济大学讲师、硕士研究生导师。致力于早期肺癌术后复发的临床和基础研究，在*American Journal of Clinical Oncology*、*Journal of Thoracic Oncology*、*Modern Pathology*等高水平期刊上，以第一/通讯作者（含共同）发表SCI论文27篇（近5年20篇，单篇最高影响因子44.544），相关成果写入中国临床肿瘤学会（CSCO）《2020 CSCO非小细胞肺癌诊疗指南》、国际肺癌研究协会（IASLC）《2017年早期肺癌诊治进展》、美国胸外科医师协会（STS）继续医学再教育CME项目（胸心外科医师必读论文）等，并被*Lancet*、*Circulation*、*Journal of the American College of Cardiology*、*American Journal of Clinical Oncology*等权威期刊引用；主持国家自然科学基金青年项目1项及省部级课题多项，入选上海市科学技术委员会"启明星计划"、上海市教育委员会"晨光计划"、上海市卫生健康委员会"医苑新星计划"等；杜克大学医学肿瘤中心Clinical　Fellow[美国胸外科学会（AATS）全额资助]；受邀赴日本呼吸器外科年会发言，并获*Journal of the American Chemical Society*旅行奖；获上海市抗癌科技一等奖（第三完成人）及上海市医学科技二等奖（第五完成人）。

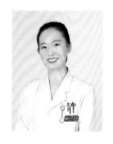

副主编：贾林沛

首都医科大学宣武医院肾内科

医学博士，首都医科大学宣武医院肾内科医师、讲师，长期从事器官衰老及衰老相关肾脏疾病方向研究，现发表SCI文章近40篇，单篇最高影响因子44.184；主持国家自然科学基金、北京市教育委员会科技一般项目等各级科研课题；入选"北京市优秀人才培育–青年骨干人才"、北京市医院管理局"青苗"人才计划；曾任SCI期刊*Annals of Translational Medicine*的专栏编辑，现任中文核心期刊《临床与病理杂志》、*Medicine International*编委，兼任30本SCI期刊审稿专家。

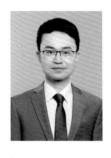

副主编：姜龙

上海交通大学附属胸科医院肺部肿瘤外科

上海交通大学附属胸科医院肺部肿瘤外科主治医师，中山大学和加州大学旧金山分校医学博士；上海市人才发展资金获得者，国际肺癌研究协会（IASLC）预防筛查早期诊断委员会委员，吴阶平医学基金会模拟医学部胸外科专业委员会青年委员，上海市生物医药行业协会精准医疗专家委员会委员；被中国临床肿瘤学会（CSCO）评选为首届"35位35岁以下最具潜力青年肿瘤医生"，广东省高层次人才评审专家，广东省基础与应用基础研究基金项目评审专家，广东省优秀毕业生。

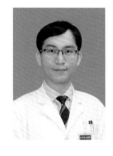

副主编：花苏榕

北京协和医院外科

医学博士，主治医师。2011年毕业于北京协和医学院（清华大学医学部）临床医学八年制（临床医学博士）并被评为当年全校毕业生代表，毕业后在北京协和医院外科工作至今。曾获北京协和医院外科技能大赛冠军、优秀员工、优秀住院医师、优秀临床带教老师等奖项和称号，目前担任《中华内分泌外科杂志》《中华消化外科杂志》《中国普通外科杂志》《临床与病理杂志》中青年编委兼审稿专家，中国研究型医院学会甲状旁腺及骨代谢疾病专业委员会委员兼秘书，中华消化外科菁英荟胰腺外科学组秘书，中国抗癌协会肿瘤微创治疗专业委员会甲状腺专业学组青年委员等。以第一负责人承担1项国家自然科学基金及多项其他科研项目，参与多项国家自然科学基金及其他研究课题。以第一作者发表SCI及核心期刊论文10余篇。以第一发明人申请及持有发明专利3项，实用新型专利8项，其中已有6项转化，累计转化金额64万元。曾参加央视、北京卫视、浙江卫视多档健康科普节目。曾获邀赴哈佛大学、芝加哥大学、香港大学等交流，并多次在国际会议上发言。

主　编：张开平

副主编：韩金鸣　　　戴晨阳　　　贾林沛　　　姜　龙　　　花苏榕

编　委：杨芳慧　　　林　瑶　　　尚炳含　　　黎少灵　　　徐小悦

丛书介绍

很高兴，由AME出版社、中南大学出版社联合出品的"AME科研时间系列医学图书"，如期与大家见面！

虽然学了4年零3个月医科，但是，仅仅做了3个月实习医生，就选择弃医了，不务正业，直到现在在做医学学术出版和传播这份工作。2015年，毕业10周年。想当医生的那份情结依旧有那么一点，有时候不经意间会触动到心底深处……

2011年4月，我和丁香园的创始人李天天一起去美国费城出差，参观了一家医学博物馆——马特博物馆（The Mütter Museum）。该博物馆隶属于费城医学院，创建于1858年，如今这里已经成为一个展出各种疾病、伤势、畸形案例，以及古代医疗器械和生物学发展的大展厅，展品逾20 000件，其中包括战争中伤者的照片、连体人的遗体、侏儒的骸骨以及人体病变结肠等。此外还有世界上独一无二的收藏，比如一个酷似肥皂的女性尸体、一个长有两个脑袋的儿童的颅骨等。该博物馆号称"Birthplace of American Medicine"。走进一个礼堂，博物馆的解说员介绍宾夕法尼亚大学医学院开学典礼都会在这个礼堂举行。当时，我忍不住问了李天天一个问题：如果当初你学医的时候，开学典礼在这样的礼堂召开的话，你会放弃做医生吗？他的回答是：不会。

2013年5月，参加《英国医学杂志》（BMJ）的一个会议，会议之后，有一个晚宴，BMJ为英国一些优秀的医疗团队颁奖，BMJ的主编和BBC电台的著名节目主持人共同主持这个年度颁奖晚宴。令我惊讶的是，BMJ给每个获奖团队的颁奖词，从未提及该团队过去几年在什么"大牛"杂志上发表过什么"大牛"论文，而是关注这些团队在某个领域提高医疗服务质量，减轻病患痛苦，降低医疗费用等方面作出的贡献。

很多朋友好奇地问我，AME是什么意思？

AME的意思就是，Academic Made Easy, Excellent and Enthusiastic。2014年9月3日，我在朋友圈贴3张图片，请大家帮忙一起从3个版本的AME宣传彩页中选出一个喜欢的。最后，上海中山医院胸外科的沈亚星医生竟然给出一个AME的"神翻译"：欲穷千里目，快乐搞学术。

AME是一个年轻的公司，拥有自己的梦想。我们的核心价值观第一条是：Patients Come First！以"科研（Research）"为主线。于是，2014年4月

24日，我们的微信公众号上线，取名为"科研时间"。"爱临床，爱科研，也爱听故事。我是科研时间，这里提供最新科研资讯，一线报道学术活动，分享科研背后的故事。用国际化视野，共同关注临床科研，相约科研时间。"希望我们的AME平台，能够推动医学学术向前进步，哪怕是一小步！

如果说酒品如人品，那么，书品更似人品。希望我们"AME科研时间系列医学图书"丛书能将临床、科研、人文三者有机结合到一起，像西餐一样，烹调出丰富的味道，搭配出一道精美的佳肴，一一呈现给各位。

汪道远
AME出版社社长

序（一）

和很多80后同龄人一样，我幼时最大的愿望是当科学家。后来，由于高考前家人离世，我的愿望便多了一个——当临床医生。所以，我捧着汇编了全国大学各专业的厚重的高考志愿填报指导书研究了好几天——哪个学校的哪个专业可以让我同时实现以上两个愿望？就这样，哈尔滨医科大学基础医学（7年制）专业进入我的视线。入学后我才知道，我们的确要学习临床医生所需学的所有课程并通过考试，也要去临床轮转实习，但我们的培养目标是做转化研究，我们不会获得临床医学学位，因此也做不了临床医生。对于临床，我依然印象深刻的是，在哈尔滨医科大学附属第二医院老年科轮转时，写病例记录写到手疼、忘食，主任还为此请我好好吃了一顿。

前两年，我有幸获得在英国帝国理工大学学习公共卫生学的机会。我选修了机器学习，考试之一是对一篇已经发表在国际某知名期刊的机器学习文章进行点评。考试前，老师详细地介绍了希望看到我们点评的思考维度。其中有一条是，希望我们去审核这篇文章有没有按照"临床预测模型建立、验证的报告规范：TRIPOD声明"来书写，哪些点遗漏了。这意味着什么？意味着这篇文章的结论可靠度和外推性究竟因此折损多少。为此，老师不仅详细地为我们介绍了什么是TRIPOD，还用许多案例让我们真正理解这个规范里每一个约束条目究竟是什么意思。

我深受触动。一些国外的优秀学校和机构早在学生的研究生阶段便开始重视、教授、普及论文的撰写规范了，而国内不少临床医生、临床医学生却因缺乏规范和系统的培训，要么弄不清病例记录和病例报告的区别，要么不知道怎么把自己手里的一份很有价值的病例以英文病例报告（case report）的方式进行撰稿发表。虽然针对病例报告如何规范撰写的指南——《病例报告指南》（CAse REport guidelines，CARE）早在2013年就发布了。

当我们AME出版社的汪道远社长告诉我，AME想要就以上现状做点事情时，我很高兴。《病例报告撰写规范CARE解读》便因此诞生了。考虑到临床工作者工作繁忙，本书从策划开始就计划做到精简和实用——最好花几小时就能读完；要有大量举例，少讲空话，要能让临床医生、临床医学生看了就会用。为此，《病例报告撰写规范CARE解读》全书仅有四个章节：第一章介绍病例报告的重要性，病例报告发表井喷和报告质量低下的现状，CARE的诞生历史，以及目前各期刊对CARE的应用情况；第二章详细解析了CARE里13个条目的含义和要求，并配备了案例说明——怎样撰写是不合格的、怎样是欠佳的、怎样是良好的；第三章介绍了大家可以在日常工作中何时、何种场景下灵活运用CARE；第四章选取了3篇已发表的代表性病例报告，用案例的方式解说为什么这些病例报告撰写得好，哪里好，哪里还可以更好。

德国哲学家、数学家Gottfried Wilhelm Leibniz说："世界上没有完全相同的两片树叶"。在个体化医疗时代，为患者制定最适合的诊疗方案变得尤为重要和充满挑战。再加之新型冠状病毒肺炎的全球大流行，病例报告的作用愈加突出。科学的螺旋式演进之旅中，我们往往先是依靠病例报告而敏锐地发现线索、提出最早的假说，然后才是验证假说。出版《病例报告撰写规范CARE解读》不只是为了规范文章的撰写，更是希望通过更规范而透明的病例报告，来帮助临床的"福尔摩斯们"更容易地揪出疾病这一"犯人"犯罪的线索、推动学术假说的提出、启发验证假说的学术研究开展，最终推动科学的螺旋式演进，使患者受益。

我想借此由衷感谢汪道远社长提出出版此书的想法。这本书的完成离不开杨芳慧女士、林瑶女士、尚炳含女士、黎少灵女士、徐小悦女士等诸多优秀的AME同事们的努力，还要特别感谢韩金鸣老师、戴晨阳老师、贾林沛老师、姜龙老师和花苏榕老师通读全书并提供宝贵建议，撰序分享对病例报告的真知灼见。

无论我幼时的两个愿望还能否实现，作为一名期刊编辑，我无比荣幸能参与对临床和学术有助益之事。此书中哪怕有一点内容能对从事科研工作、临床工作的读者有一丝帮助或启发，我便觉自己非无用之人并将为此更加乐此不疲。

是为序。

张开平

2022年1月26日于杭州

序（二）

最近收到了合作者美国Mayo Clinic神经内科Zbigniew K. Wszolek教授的邮件（我们因共同关注一种神经系统罕见疾病而相识多年）。在邮件中，教授提到他作为多本SCI期刊的审稿人，最近审阅了许多篇来自中国的相关病例报告，并勉励我们留学回国后继续关注该罕见疾病，与国际同行一道积极探索可能的治疗方案。

的确，临床医生不断总结一些罕见疾病的临床实践经验和教训，并通过病例报告的形式发表在国际学术期刊上，可以促进国内外同行间的交流。病例报告往往预示着新的疾病，新的诊疗手段，易被忽视的症状体征和不良反应，可以为临床医生今后开启高质量观察类研究或随机对照研究提供切入点。然而，英文病例报告的撰写和我们日常病程记录差异很大。国内部分临床医生缺乏系统性和规范性的科研培训，撰写并发表英文病例报告并非易事，且病例报告的最终发表也并不仅仅依赖于病例的罕见程度。

为了促进病例报告的规范化，多学科专家共同制定的《病例报告指南》（CARE）应运而生。CARE结构化的条目可以提示作者撰写病例报告时需要重点考虑的条目，进而帮助作者写好一份病例报告。笔者作为多本SCI期刊审稿人，也会按照CARE条目对相关病例报告文章批判性地提出审稿意见，如提醒作者以时间轴的形式记录重要临床信息和治疗节点。目前，越来越多的期刊根据CARE对病例报告类型的稿件进行规范化约束，有的临床小伙伴直到期刊编辑发来退稿信，让其在投稿系统补充材料里上传CARE清单时，还搞不清楚CARE是什么以及如何填写清单。

《病例报告撰写规范CARE解读》这本书凝聚了AME出版社编辑们的心血，对CARE的条目进行了深入的解读，内容全面详实。编辑们分享了处理稿件的心得，并结合AME出版社发表的病例报告实例对CARE的条目进行了细致的讲解。目前市面上尚未有类似的出版物。我相信《病例报告撰写规范CARE解读》的出版，会在一定程度上促进病例报告更规范地报告。

为此，我欣然接受AME出版社的作序邀请。同时，把《病例报告撰写规范CARE解读》这本书推荐给各位读者，特别是专业型学位的研究生和正在接受住院医师规范化培训的年轻医生，相信大家都能够从中受益。

韩金鸣
2022年春节于北京

序（三）

2022年3月以来，奥密克戎变异株突袭了整个上海，医学界普遍认为我们面对的是一种全新的病毒。面对种种未知，作为最早一批医疗救援队的成员，我踏入方舱医院正式开展工作。

工作的前几天，令人感到无所适从的是，我所面对的不再是熟悉的胸部疾病患者，现有知识储备无法让我从容面对各种合并慢性病、高龄、精神疾病的感染者。事实上，在疫情期间的科室病例讨论中，我们原有的患者在治疗上也面临着大量挑战。例如，肺移植前受体是否需要疫苗接种？移植后受体感染"新冠肺炎"的具体治疗方案等。大量的新问题必须从文献中获取答案。令人遗憾的是，海量的文献告诉了我们前后矛盾的结论（如移植患者接种疫苗的必要性）抑或是缺乏重要且基本的临床信息（感染的病毒株类型）等。因此，前人总结病例报告形成的经验最终并没有帮助到我们。

随着进入疫情的后期，大家已深深意识到，我们面对的奥密克戎变异株不仅仅是一个医疗问题。第一，涉及面广。在中国香港，新型冠状病毒在3个月内感染了约15%的人群，这个数据远超发病率位居各种疾病前列的肺癌（每年约0.5‰）。第二，缺乏人群特异性。笔者在方舱医院内接诊过1岁的幼儿，也接诊过99岁的高龄老年人；有免疫缺陷状态的患者，也有晚期肿瘤患者。可见，这已经是影响到每个人的公共卫生问题，而公共卫生政策制定的基础是医学科学家们最终发表的病例报告。这再一次提醒我们，病例报告的撰写容不得半点懈怠，它最终将影响到每个人。

病例报告作为传播交流临床实践经验的重要载体，如何进行规范和统一，完成经验的传递呢？正如本书所重点介绍的《病例报告指南》（CARE），其是按照病例报告写作框架制定的结构化自查清单，它使得最后的论文有据可循，既突出其重点，又兼顾细节，并精准无误。当然最大的作用是，它让我们的研究报告成为高质量的临床证据，精准地指导实践，解决我们的临床困境。

再等等，疫情的阴霾终将散去，临床疑惑也会因为高质量的病例报告而豁然开朗。

戴晨阳
2022年5月9日于上海市杨浦区共青路方舱医院

序（四）

解读CARE，让病例报告撰写不再迷茫

刚刚开始做临床医生的时候，我总是信心满满，自以为熟读了课本就可以有恃无恐，然而随着工作时间的延长，我清楚地认识到，临床疾病的诊治并没有固定的程序化流程可以遵循。常见疾病可能有罕见表现，而罕见疾病也可能表现为若干常见症状的"随机"拼凑，让人摸不着头脑。诚然，现代医学是科学的重要分支，追求客观性、普适性，然而依据经验积累构建的诊疗思维仍然是临床工作的主体。但相较于浩瀚如星辰的庞大疾病谱，医生在短短几十年的临床生涯中所见的病例是十分有限的，我们需要借助更多的"他人之事"作为"我事之师"。这时，病例报告就成了传递临床经验的最佳载体。

纵观医学史，临床病例报告应该是最早期的医学传播形式之一，其目的是以文字为载体，将某种罕见疾病的临床表现、诊疗经验及转归情况广泛传递，以推动临床医学进步。临床工作者对军团菌肺炎、IgG4相关性疾病、艾滋病等大众耳熟能详的疾病最初的认知都是通过临床病例报告呈现的。后续随着临床诊疗需求扩大，一些常见疾病的罕见症状、新颖的治疗方案、失败的经验教训也逐步成为临床病例报告的丰富题材。

记得内科轮转时期，我最喜欢的课外书就是《北京协和医院内科大查房》，里面"烧脑"的病例和教授们精彩的分析让我对这套书爱不释手。后来，我开始关注《新英格兰医学杂志》（*The New England Journal of Medicine*，*NEJM*）中的"临床病例"一栏，对其每次推出的新病例，我都仔细啃下并慢慢消化，从中受益良多。现在回过头去看，优秀的临床病例报告不是症状和诊疗的简单罗列，而是严谨、缜密临床思维方式的体现，它指导我们如何抽丝剥茧找到关键问题，如何以科学的眼光看待疾病发展，以及如何利用临床科研和基础科研成果指导诊疗。因此，一份逻辑清晰、内容优质、写作规范的临床病例报告真的太重要了。

那么，怎样才能写出优秀的临床病例报告呢？这一直是困扰国内很多临床医生的问题。我们国家拥有庞大的诊疗体量和丰富的病例资源，我们在临床实践中经常能遇到很多高质量病例，但大部分临床工作者却对临床病例报告写作这种西方医学"舶来品"不得要领，面临着"病例好、发表难"的困境。为了规范病例报告写作，使更多的优秀病例能够发表，《病例报告指南》

（CARE）诞生了，CARE以逐条提示的结构化条目指引临床研究者完成一份规范的病例报告，同时方便作者自查。

我第一份英文病例报告的顺利发表也得益于CARE的指导。最开始写作时，我也不得要领，难以表达病例临床诊疗的精髓，于是编辑部要求我先对照CARE自查修改。虽然结构化条目逻辑清晰明了，但作为病例报告写作的初学者，我在分析CARE过程中难免有所偏差，最终几经返修才得以发表。当时我就想，要是有一本CARE的解读书在手就太好了。因此，当我从张开平老师手中收到这本《病例报告撰写规范CARE解读》时，我着实欣喜万分。在从北京东四环开往西四环的地铁上，我用一小时的时间一口气通读了全部内容。这本汇聚了AME出版社编辑们心血的小册子，以通俗而严谨的语言详细分析了CARE的各项要求，也解答了我当初的所有疑问。作为AME出版社的老朋友，我知道他们一直以解决临床科研工作者实际需求为出发点，做实事、做好事，而这内容精致、"干货"满满的《病例报告撰写规范CARE解读》正是AME出版社工作者们秉承初心的体现。

最后，希望每一位读者在这本书中有所收获，也希望我们国家有更多的优秀病例诊疗经验得以在世界上推广，期待医学不断进步，实现我们当初的诺言——除人类之病痛，助健康之完美！

贾林沛

2022年1月28日于北京

序（五）

最初与AME出版社结缘，是笔者在旧金山接受博士联合培养之时。从担任AME出版社旗下期刊的专栏编辑（Section Editor）开始，笔者在AME出版社搭建的平台上开始结识业内的专家与同道，也有幸结识了本书的主编张开平总监。此后，在旧金山锡安山（Mount Zion）、广州东风东路、杭州解放路、上海淮海西路、北京车公庄大街，笔者在经历不同生活与工作环境的同时，也与国内外同道共同见证了AME出版社逐步成为国内生物医学类较为出色的学术出版与交流平台的过程。可以说，AME出版社"穷理以致其知，反躬以践其实"，为"把论文写在祖国的大地上"，解决中国学术期刊的"卡脖子"问题走出了一条可行之路。

病例报告应该是每一位医学科研工作者都非常熟悉的论文类型。具有言简意赅、内容翔实、视角独特、引人入胜的特殊魅力，也是相当多学者迈入学术殿堂的第一步。包括《新英格兰医学杂志》（*The New England Journal of Medicine*，*NEJM*）在内的众多顶级学术期刊也都为这一论文类型提供了展示舞台。一个个经典的病例报告，为我们展示着医学发展史上的一座座里程碑，有内科医生首次报道的疾病，有外科医生独创的术式，也有病理科医生全新的发现。病例报告，既是学术的呈现，也是历史的记录。

但是，正如本书中展示的数据，病例报告的发文数量逐年攀升，但报告质量却不尽如人意，难以为临床研究设计提供有效依据，也难以精准地指导临床实践。本书的一众编者，从细节处着手，旨在通过介绍与解读《病例报告指南》（*CARE*），助推研究者更规范地撰写与发表病例报告。

开局关系全局，起步决定后势。病例报告可能是许多医学科研工作者的论文"首秀"，而如何做好这个开局"首秀"，迈好学术生涯第一步，对于医学科研工作者来说至关重要。做学问是发现事物、探索事物本质的过程，是"求是"的过程。对待学术首先要有一个端正的态度，才能进一步把研究做好。如何严谨地做学术，关系着能够到达的学术高度。有多严谨的治学态度，就有多高的学术水平。希望读者通过本书以及AME科研时间系列医学图书，系好学术发展道路上第一颗"扣子"，遵守学术规范，严谨治学，成为负责的学术接班人。

是为序！

姜龙

2022年初春于上海

序（六）

近年来，医学界的科研评价体系正在从"唯文章论、唯论著论"逐渐走向多元化，开始强调科研对临床的实际帮助意义。医生不再一味地追求发表文章的数量，也不再一味地追求发表论著，因而得以更多地回归临床工作。过去因为被引用率低而备受冷落的病例报告，由于其更符合医生日常的病例书写习惯、更贴近医生的日常诊疗工作、更有利于普通医生之间的经验传播、更有助于临床思维训练而日益受到重视。

在医学知识共同体的发展中，理论性的结构化知识作为基石固然非常重要，但这类知识的产生需要大量的数据、严谨的分析，并不适合所有医生。一方面，不是每一位医生都具备丰富的资源、较高的统计水平与良好的论文写作能力；另一方面，也不是每一位读者都愿意花费较长时间，带着批判性思维去反复阅读一篇严谨的论著。大家逐渐发现，在各种医学会议上，病例讨论的观众参与度高、互动性强，通常比长篇论著更受读者的欢迎（虽然不容易产生引用）。

论著的行文模式，是基于对大样本的统计和分析，其重视对数据的统计和对客观规律的分析，却难以触及患者的心理、家庭以及社会因素。而病例报告虽然难以揭示宏观的整体规律，但在对具体问题的分析上，可以结合患者的心理、社会因素，进行更加深入而个性化的讨论。从医学模式的角度看，生物医学模式的建立使得医学进入了现代科学的范畴，医学知识的迅速积累和医学技术的不断革新，催生了循证医学的大发展，大量的论著和证据推动指南不断更新，使得疾病诊疗的成功率逐渐提升。但若把重心过多地放在了对抗"病"，而忽略了"人"的因素，则容易陷入"技术至上"的误区。现在广为倡导的生物–心理–社会模式，在强调做好生物医学治疗的同时，重视患者的心理和社会属性。而目前的论著范式每次只能关注一个点，尚难以体现生物–心理–社会模式的整体性思路。

此外，即使把心理和社会因素放在一边，仅考虑生物医学范畴，循证医学的发展也达到了瓶颈。基于"干预方法A通过通路B，影响结局C在疾病D中的应用/机制"的研究模式，越来越难以回答现实中"多种干预和药物共用，多个脏器功能结局要考虑，且多种疾病共存"的情况。未来无论是中国还是世界，都注定处于一个老龄化的时代，这是一个多种疾患共病、多种价值取向共存的时代。患者不再单纯因某一个病来就诊，而是带着多种基础病及个人和家庭的需求来就诊；医生也不仅仅要诊疗眼前的疾病，还要考虑患者的既往史，往往需要请其他科室会诊，或者启动多学科诊疗模式（MDT），甚至越来越多地被要求考虑患者的心理因素、家庭关系和价值观。因此，根据单个患者的情况进行MDT讨论，从而为其制定个体化诊疗方案，这在未来将会越来越普遍。而目前这个领域最常用的学术交流方式就是病例报告。

需要注意的是，写一篇病例报告绝不等于照搬临床病例，更不只是记流水账。病例报告源于病例，而高于病例，要遵循2013年发布的《病例报告指南》（CARE）及2017年发布的CARE解释与说明性文件。对作者来说，CARE会提出灵魂的拷问：是否考虑了患者的观点？知情同意是否完整？患者对干预的依从性和耐受性如何？有没有回避治疗中的不良事件？对广大读者来说，病例报告要有启发性，要有教育意义，要对临床诊疗思路或者方法的改良有所助益。帮助更多医生朋友们写好病例报告正是本书的目的。

本书对CARE进行了解读。从期刊编辑的视角，以幽默诙谐的语言，提供了CARE的使用说明书，不仅有常见不良病例报告的问题和解决方案，还附上了优秀病例报告供大家借鉴参考。对于初次撰写病例报告的年轻医生来说，相信会有不小的帮助。

AME（意为Academic Made Easy, Excellent and Enthusiastic）有一个中文神翻译——"欲穷千里目，快乐搞学术"。那么，在我们紧张的临床工作之余，还有什么比读到一篇精彩的病例报告更让人惬意的呢？

花苏榕

目　录

第一章　《病例报告指南》：让病例报告更规范、透明、有据可循
杨芳慧 ·· 1

第二章　如何写好一份病例报告：《病例报告指南》条目解析
张开平 ·· 9

第三章　"治疗"病例报告报告质量不佳：《病例报告指南》使用说明书
林瑶 ·· 30

第四章　病例报告示例
尚炳含 ·· 36

I

第一章 《病例报告指南》：让病例报告更规范、透明、有据可循

　　在人类对抗疾病的漫长科学研究和临床诊治之旅中，病例报告就像一名"哨兵"，总是冲在最前面，告知我们前方是万丈深渊还是绿洲良田。而《病例报告指南》（*CAse REport guidelines*，*CARE*），便是这名"哨兵"手里的工具、"宝箱"，帮助其有据可循，使其报告既要点突出，又详尽无遗且精准无误。

一、病例报告：科学研究与临床诊治的"哨兵"

　　20世纪60年代前，沙利度胺因被认为比巴比妥类药物更安全而在全球40多个国家中被推荐使用，以减轻孕妇妊娠晨吐反应。而在1961年，来自Distillers Company（Biochemicals）Ltd.的Hayman致信给*British Medical Journal*（*BMJ*）[1]：两例病例报告提示，沙利度胺可能对怀孕初期胎儿产生有害影响。在进一步调查之前，该公司决定从市场上撤出其所有含有沙利度胺的制剂。之后，*The Lancet*期刊的病例报告[2-4]也证实沙利度胺可能与新生儿先天畸形有关。沙利度胺的召回，使全世界难计其数的婴幼儿免遭不幸。21世纪，一篇病例报告[5]的出现也让世界各地罹患血管瘤的婴幼儿因普萘洛尔药物有了更多治疗的可能。

　　病例报告，顾名思义，是"一份详细的叙述，描述一个或多个患者所经历的医学问题，以达到医学、科学或教育的目的"[6]。病例报告能在识别不良和

有益的影响中发挥作用，并能帮助识别新的疾病、常见疾病的不寻常形式以及罕见疾病的表现[7]。病例报告还可为未来的研究提出假设，指导个体化治疗，促进不同文化间医疗教育和服务的交流[8-9]。

二、病例报告的数量井喷与堪忧的报告质量

正是因为上述病例报告的重要价值，越来越多期刊将关注点放在病例报告上。专注报道病例的*Journal of Medical Case Reports*于2007年1月由BioMed Central正式创刊[10]。次年，BioMed Central又创办了同样专注于发表病例报告的*Cases Journal*[11]。同年，*BMJ*也创办了病例报告期刊*BMJ Case Reports*[12]。这些期刊为我们带来了病例报告的新视角，例如，*Cases Journal*会接收患者提交的文章。这3本专注报道病例报告的期刊的诞生，促使了更多发表病例报告的期刊的创建。2018年、2019年和2020年这3年发表病例报告的期刊总数分别达3 515种、3 682种与3 663种（数据来源：Web of Science，2021年8月16日）。不仅如此，病例报告本身的发文数量也逐年攀升。Web of Science数据库显示，2018年、2019年与2020年的病例报告发表量分别为29 357篇、32 370篇与37 998篇。

病例报告发表数量虽然大，但这些文章的报告质量却参差不齐。一项研究评估了来自4家同行评审的急诊医学期刊的1 316份病例报告，发现超过一半的文章没有提供与主要治疗相关的信息，而这些信息可以帮助增加文章的透明度和可复制性[13]。在没有报告准则的情况下撰写的病例报告往往不够严谨，难以进行数据汇总分析，难以为临床研究设计提供有效依据，也难以精准地指导临床实践[13-14]。

三、解决报告不规范的方案：遵循报告指南

随着人们逐渐意识到规范、全面和透明的病例报告的重要性，针对各类研究的报告指南应运而生。过去20余年里，由方法学家、医学期刊编辑和医疗保健专家等组成的多学科小组已经制定出一系列报告指南，以此提高论文的报告质量[15-16]。

报告指南是期刊对作者要求的补充说明，它们通常采用清单的形式，提供关于如何撰写研究报告的结构化建议。制定这些指南时通常遵循明确的方法，系统检索相关证据和共识的过程是制定报告指南的关键环节[17]。如针对2组平行随机对照试验的《临床试验报告的统一标准》（*Consolidated Standards of Reporting Trials*，CONSORT），包含25个条目和1个流程图，是第一个被广泛应

用于数百种医学期刊的报告指南[18]。已有证据表明，期刊采用CONSORT指南能提高随机试验的报告完整性[19]。

CONSORT指南的出现促进了许多其他报告指南的制定。如针对观察性研究的《加强流行病学中观察性研究报告质量声明》[20]（Strengthening the Reporting of Observational studies in Epidemiology，STROBE），针对系统评价和荟萃分析的《系统评价和Meta分析优先报告条目》[21]（Preferred Reporting Items for Systematic Reviews and Meta-Analyses，PRISMA），以及针对诊断准确性研究的《诊断准确性研究报告规范》（Standards for Reporting of Diagnostic Accuracy，STARD）等[22]。在撰写本章节时，加强生物医学研究报告质量和透明度（Enhancing the Quality and Transparency Of health Research，EQUATOR）网站[23]已收录超过400种生物医学研究报告指南，并同步展示众多研发中的报告指南。

四、解决病例报告撰写不规范：*CARE*

病例发表量的逐年递增，以及病例报告在教育、临床研究与临床实践中的重要作用，促使了专门针对病例报告的报告指南的诞生。

2011年，CARE制定小组由临床医生、研究人员和期刊编辑组成，计划通过三阶段共识过程来制定病例报告的报告指南，包括：①会前文献回顾、访谈，形成病例报告的初始报告条目；②召开面对面共识会议，起草报告指南；③会后反馈和试点测试，然后确定《病例报告指南》。最终，CARE共包含13个条目。这些条目在2013年国际同行评审和生物医学出版大会上被提出，得到了多家医学期刊的认可，并于同年在7本期刊上发表[24-30]，分别为*BMJ Case Reports*、*Global Advances in Health and Medicine*、*Deutsches Arzteblatt International*、*Journal of Clinical Epidemiology*、*Journal of Medical Case Reports*、*Journal of Dietary Supplements*与*Headache*，还被翻译成多种语言[31]。2017年，Riley等在*Journal of Clinical Epidemiology*上进一步发表了CARE的解释与说明文件，对CARE每个条目进行详细解释并提供示例，更加具体地指导病例报告的撰写[32]。

此外，Sun等在*Journal of Clinical Epidemiology*上针对病例报告的透明规范报告也提出了12个条目[33]，但由于其仅由3人制定且缺乏像CARE这样严格系统的制定过程，最终没有获得世界范围内的广泛认可和使用。

CARE（图1-1）为撰写病例报告提供了一个框架，使用者还可根据具体情况进行调整，以包括不同专业的具体信息。

CARE case report guidelines

CARE Checklist of information to include when writing a case report

Topic	Item	Checklist item description	Reported on Line
Title	1	The diagnosis or intervention of primary focus followed by the words "case report"	
Key Words	2	2 to 5 key words that identify diagnoses or interventions in this case report, including "case report"	
Abstract (no references)	3a	Introduction: What is unique about this case and what does it add to the scientific literature?	
	3b	Main symptoms and/or important clinical findings	
	3c	The main diagnoses, therapeutic interventions, and outcomes	
	3d	Conclusion—What is the main "take-away" lesson(s) from this case?	
Introduction	4	One or two paragraphs summarizing why this case is unique (**may include references**)	
Patient Information	5a	De-identified patient specific information.	
	5b	Primary concerns and symptoms of the patient.	
	5c	Medical, family, and psycho-social history including relevant genetic information	
	5d	Relevant past interventions with outcomes	
Clinical Findings	6	Describe significant physical examination (PE) and important clinical findings.	
Timeline	7	Historical and current information from this episode of care organized as a timeline	
Diagnostic Assessment	8a	Diagnostic testing (such as PE, laboratory testing, imaging, surveys).	
	8b	Diagnostic challenges (such as access to testing, financial, or cultural)	
	8c	Diagnosis (including other diagnoses considered)	
	8d	Prognosis (such as staging in oncology) where applicable	
Therapeutic Intervention	9a	Types of therapeutic intervention (such as pharmacologic, surgical, preventive, self-care)	
	9b	Administration of therapeutic intervention (such as dosage, strength, duration)	
	9c	Changes in therapeutic intervention (with rationale)	
Follow-up and Outcomes	10a	Clinician and patient-assessed outcomes (if available)	
	10b	Important follow-up diagnostic and other test results	
	10c	Intervention adherence and tolerability (How was this assessed?)	
	10d	Adverse and unanticipated events	
Discussion	11a	A scientific discussion of the strengths AND limitations associated with this case report	
	11b	Discussion of the relevant medical literature **with references**.	
	11c	The scientific rationale for any conclusions (including assessment of possible causes)	
	11d	The primary "take-away" lessons of this case report (without references) in a one paragraph conclusion	
Patient Perspective	12	The patient should share their perspective in one to two paragraphs on the treatment(s) they received	
Informed Consent	13	Did the patient give informed consent? Please provide if requested	Yes ☐ No ☐

图1–1 《病例报告指南》（*CARE*）条目[24]

五、*CARE*的官方认可与执行落差

*CARE*自2013年发表以来，得到了作者、期刊编辑和同行评议人员的广泛认可。*CARE*官网（https://www.care-statement.org）数据显示，目前*CARE*已获得至少126本期刊的明确肯定与采纳，还被EQUATOR网站收录并被置于网站首页重点推荐。

虽然*CARE*在表面上得到众多期刊认可，但绝大多数期刊并未强制要求作者按*CARE*撰写病例报告。Calvache等发现，*The Journal of the American Medical Association*（*JAMA*）、*The Lancet*、*The New England Journal of Medicine*（*NEJM*）及专注发表病例报告的*BMJ Case Reports*这4本知名期刊中，仅*BMJ Case Reports*与*JAMA*在作者须知中明确要求使用*CARE*，而*The Lancet*与*NEJM*并未提及*CARE*[34]。另外，我们查询2020年病例报告发表量排名前10的期刊官网后发现，这些期刊也并未都强制要求作者使用*CARE*（表1–1）。在这10本期刊中，只有*Medicine*、*BMJ Case Reports*与*Clinical Case Report* 3本期刊明确要求使用*CARE*。

表1-1　2020年病例报告发表量排名前10的期刊（Web of Science）要求使用CARE的情况

期刊名	是否强制要求使用CARE	病例报告发表数	占比*/%
Cureus	否	1 899	5.0
International Journal of Surgery Case Reports	否	1 064	2.8
Medicine	是	983	2.6
BMJ Case Reports	是	575	1.5
World Neurosurgery	否	562	1.5
The American Journal of Case Reports	否	546	1.4
World Journal of Clinical Cases	否	457	1.2
Clinical Case reports	是	359	0.9
Radiology Case Reports	否	348	0.9
Journal of Surgical Case Reports	否	325	0.9

注：*该期刊在2020年发表的病例报告占该年所有期刊发表的病例报告（37 998篇）的百分比。

正是因为期刊表面上对CARE的认可和执行上的巨大落差，病例报告的报告质量才有很大进步空间。Eldawlatly等评估了2013—2017年发表在*Saudi Journal of Anaesthesia*上的病例报告的完整性，发现患者对病例发表的观点（CARE条目12）和知情同意（CARE条目13）亟需改善[35]。Dragnev等发现，以孤立性脾脏转移为研究对象的55篇病例报告中没有1篇完全遵循CARE，所有病例报告均未报告患者观点（CARE条目12），只有2份病例报告列出了时间轴（CARE条目7）[36]。

六、未来之路：给"哨兵"配备工具，学会如何用好工具

CARE的执行不佳及病例报告堪忧的报告质量，促进了更多针对病例报告的报告指南的制定。撰写本章节时，在EQUATOR网站检索到病例报告相关的报告指南有32种，这还并未包括那些正在研发的报告指南。

报告指南真的越多越好吗？我们不断研发新的报告指南，究竟是因为目前没有适用的报告指南来规范稿件，还是因为我们没有用好已有的报告指南？

这20多年间，我们从没有报告指南到拥有超过400种报告指南，从病例报告的无据可循到有了CARE的有据可循，我们已经成功地让病例报告这个"哨兵"手持CARE这一绝佳工具。未来，我们更需要做的是给每个"哨兵"准确

配备应有的工具，并学会怎么用好这个工具。如此，"哨兵"便可变成"精兵强将"，可以既要点突出，又详尽无遗且精准无误地向我们报告："前方2公里有敌军3 000名，辎重充沛，其中重型枪械1 000把，轻型2 000把，粮草10车，预计今夜戌时进入我方射程，请指示。"

　　相对应地，这则消息或许是一个不错的开始：2019年10月，AME出版社发布声明，旗下60余本期刊均要求作者在投递病例报告时必须同时递交填写完成的CARE清单[37]。

参考文献

[1]　Hayman DJ. Withdrawal of Thalidomide ("Distaval")[J]. Br Med J, 1961, 2: 1499.

[2]　Mcbride WG. Thalidomide and Congenital Abnormalities[J]. Lancet, 1961, 278(7216): 1358.

[3]　Lenz W, Pfeiffer RA, Kosenow W, et al. Thalidomide and Congenital Abnormalities[J]. Lancet, 1962, 279(7219): 45-46.

[4]　SPEIRS AL. Thalidomide and congenital abnormalities[J]. Lancet, 1962, 1(7224): 303-305.

[5]　Sans V, de la Roque ED, Berge J, et al. Propranolol for severe infantile hemangiomas: follow-up report[J]. Pediatrics, 2009, 124(3): e423-e431.

[6]　Porta M. A Dictionary of Epidemiology[M]. New York: Oxford University Press, 2014: 376.

[7]　Hauben M, Aronson JK. Gold standards in pharmacovigilance: the use of definitive anecdotal reports of adverse drug reactions as pure gold and high-grade ore[J]. Drug Saf, 2007, 30(8): 645-655.

[8]　Jenicek M. Clinical case reporting in evidence-based medicine[M]. New York: Oxford University Press, 2001.

[9]　Riley D. Case reports in the era of clinical trials[J]. Glob Adv Health Med, 2013, 2(2): 10-11.

[10]　Kidd M, Hubbard C. Introducing journal of medical case reports[J]. J Med Case Rep, 2007, 1: 1.

[11]　Smith R. Why do we need Cases Journal?[J]. Cases J, 2008, 1(1): 1.

[12]　BMJ Case Reports. About[EB/OL]. [2021-08-15]. https://casereports.bmj.com/pages/about/.

[13]　Richason TP, Paulson SM, Lowenstein SR, et al. Case reports describing treatments in the emergency medicine literature: missing and misleading information[J]. BMC Emerg Med, 2009, 9: 10.

[14]　Kaszkin-Bettag M, Hildebrandt W. Case reports on cancer therapies: the urgent need to improve the reporting quality[J]. Glob Adv Health Med, 2012, 1(2): 8-10.

[15]　Moher D, Weeks L, Ocampo M, et al. Describing reporting guidelines for health research: a systematic review[J]. J Clin Epidemiol, 2011, 64(7): 718-742.

[16]　Simera I, Moher D, Hoey J, et al. A catalogue of reporting guidelines for health research[J]. Eur J Clin Invest, 2010, 40(1): 35-53.

[17] Murphy MK，Black NA，Lamping DL，et al. Consensus development methods, and their use in clinical guideline development[J]. Health Technol Assess，1998，2(3)：i-iv，1-88.

[18] Schulz KF，Altman DG，Moher D，et al. CONSORT 2010 statement：updated guidelines for reporting parallel group randomized trials[J]. Ann Intern Med，2010，152(11)：726-732.

[19] Turner L，Shamseer L，Altman DG，et al. Does use of the CONSORT Statement impact the completeness of reporting of randomised controlled trials published in medical journals? A Cochrane review[J]. Syst Rev，2012，1：60.

[20] von Elm E，Altman DG，Egger M，et al. Strengthening the Reporting of Observational Studies in Epidemiology (STROBE) statement：guidelines for reporting observational studies[J]. BMJ，2007，335(7624)：806-808.

[21] Moher D，Liberati A，Tetzlaff J，et al. Preferred reporting items for systematic reviews and meta-analyses：the PRISMA statement[J]. PLoS Med，2009，6(7)：e1000097.

[22] Bossuyt PM，Reitsma JB，Bruns DE，et al. Towards complete and accurate reporting of studies of diagnostic accuracy：the STARD initiative[J]. BMJ，2003，326(7379)：41-44.

[23] Simera I，Altman DG，Moher D，et al. Guidelines for reporting health research：the EQUATOR network's survey of guideline authors[J]. PLoS Med，2008，5(6)：e139.

[24] Gagnier JJ，Kienle G，Altman DG，et al. The CARE guidelines：consensus-based clinical case reporting guideline development[J]. BMJ Case Rep，2013，2013：bcr2013201554.

[25] Gagnier JJ，Kienle G，Altman DG，et al. The CARE Guidelines：Consensus-based Clinical Case Reporting Guideline Development[J]. Glob Adv Health Med，2013，2(5)：38-43.

[26] Gagnier JJ，Riley D，Altman DG，et al. The CARE guidelines：consensus-based clinical case reporting guideline development[J]. Dtsch Arztebl Int，2013，110(37)：603-608.

[27] Gagnier JJ，Kienle G，Altman DG，et al. The CARE guidelines：consensus-based clinical case report guideline development[J]. J Clin Epidemiol，2014，67(1)：46-51.

[28] Gagnier JJ，Kienle G，Altman DG，et al. The CARE guidelines：consensus-based clinical case report guideline development[J]. J Med Case Rep，2013，7：223.

[29] Gagnier JJ，Kienle G，Altman DG，et al. The CARE guidelines：consensus-based clinical case report guideline development[J]. J Diet Suppl，2013，10(4)：381-390.

[30] Gagnier JJ，Kienle G，Altman DG，et al. The CARE guidelines：consensus-based clinical case reporting guideline development[J]. Headache，2013，53(10)：1541-1547.

[31] SWIHM. Resources[EB/OL]. [2021-08-15]. https://swihm.com/resources/.

[32] Riley DS，Barber MS，Kienle GS，et al. CARE guidelines for case reports：explanation and elaboration document[J]. J Clin Epidemiol，2017，89：218-235.

[33] Sun GH，Aliu O，Hayward RA. Open-access electronic case report journals：the rationale for case report guidelines[J]. J Clin Epidemiol，2013，66(10)：1065-1070.

[34] Calvache JA，Vera-Montoya M，Ordoñez D，et al. Completeness of reporting of case reports in high-impact medical journals[J]. Eur J Clin Invest，2020，50(4)：e13215.

[35] Eldawlatly A，Alsultan D，Al Dammas F，et al. Adaptation of CARE (CAse REport) guidelines on published case reports in the Saudi Journal of Anesthesia[J]. Saudi J Anaesth，2018，12(3)：446-449.

[36] Dragnev NC，Wong SL. Do we CARE about the quality of case reports? A systematic assessment[J]. J Surg Res，2018，231：428-433.

[37] Editorial Office. Application of the CARE guideline as reporting standard in the AME Case Reports[J]. AME Case Rep，2019，3：47.

作者：杨芳慧，AME出版社

审核修订：张开平，AME出版社

校对：林瑶，AME出版社

　　　尚炳含，AME出版社

第二章　如何写好一份病例报告：《病例报告指南》条目解析

通过第一章，我们已经了解病例报告的重要性和使用《病例报告指南》（CARE）改善报告质量的重要性。那么，在CARE的具体使用中，清单各个条目的报告情况如何呢？Seguel-Moraga等评估2008—2018年201篇牙科领域的病例报告后发现，各条目报告情况不佳，报告频率最低的3个是时间轴（条目7）、患者观点（条目12）、知情同意（条目13）[1]。Park等评估了827篇病例报告后发现，报告严重不足的有诊断挑战（条目8b）、患者观点（条目12）、知情同意（条目13）、干预依从性和耐受性（条目10c），以及不良事件（条目10d）[2]。另外，笔者从2019年审核过的300多篇病例中提取了105篇各个条目"显示"已报告的病例报告。经分析后发现，这些声称按CARE各个条目报告的病例报告中，徒有其名的情况普遍存在。

所以，我们有必要理解CARE的各条目，这样才能运用好这一写好病例报告的绝佳工具。

一、CARE条目结构

CARE的条目共13个大类别，如第一章图1-1所示，分别是题目（title）、关键词（key words）、摘要（abstract）、引言（introduction）、患者信息（patient information）、临床发现（clinical findings）、时间轴（timeline）、诊断评估（diagnostic assessment）、治疗干预（therapeutic intervention）、随访和结局（follow-up and outcomes）、讨论（discussion）、患者观点（patient perspective）和知情同意（informed consent）。可以看出，*CARE*基本就是按照一篇病例报告的成文顺序来划定结构的。我们在成文时，是否完全按照这样的顺序均可。无论怎样，这个框架可以给病例报告的撰写提供非常好的思路和脉络，并提醒我们不要忘记撰写哪些重要事项。所以它既是一个好的撰写框架，也是一份很好的自查清单。

二、*CARE*条目解析

下面，我们就*CARE*的每个条目展开解析，并通过案例来说明，怎样的报告算到位，怎样的报告算欠佳。

（一）*CARE*条目1——标题

写明最初的诊断或干预关注点，其后加上"case report"。

条目1传达的报告思路其实就是大家熟知的PICOS：P——population，什么样的研究人群/对象/疾病；I——intervention，做了什么干预；C——control，对照是什么；O——outcome，结局是什么；S——study design，研究设计类型是什么。

不良报告示范[3]：

Neuroimaging manifestations of epidermal nevus syndrome

解析：从这个标题可以知道文章的研究对象P为表皮痣综合征，也知道文章的关注点是"神经影像学表现"。但如果只读标题，我们很难知晓这是一篇病例报告，笔者甚至误以为是综述。

欠佳报告示范[4]：

Surgical treatment of ascending aorta floating thrombus in a patient with recent SARS-CoV-2 infection

解析：这个标题比上一个好很多，主要在于"a patient"的表述，虽然没有明说是病例报告，但是能一眼看出是病例报告。这个标题也同时覆盖到了诊断和治疗两个点：感染SARS–CoV–2的患者的升主动脉浮动血栓问题和手术治疗问题。如果加入诊断挑战或者治疗结果，并且加上直白的"a case report"，这个标题会更好。

良好报告示范[5]：

Pembrolizumab-induced myocarditis in a patient with malignant mesothelioma: plasma exchange as a successful emerging therapy——case report

解析:这个标题是按照PICOS思路来拟定的,传达含义精准全面。既说明了P是帕博利珠单抗诱导的恶性间皮瘤患者的心肌炎,说清了I是血浆交换,也告知了O——治疗成功了,还让读者一眼就知道S是一则病例报告。并非所有病例报告都必须按这样的方式报告,作者还需要结合期刊的要求来综合考虑。

(二)CARE条目2——关键词

2~5个点明该病例报告的诊断或干预的关键词,包括"case report"。

关键词的拟定也可以按照PICOS思路展开,关键词和标题相对应,实际上也是标题中的核心词。例如,对于上一则"良好报告示范"案例,就可以从这些词中选取关键词:case report,pembrolizumab,myocarditis,malignant mesothelioma,plasma exchange。需要特别提醒的是,勿忘case report这个关键词。

(三)CARE条目3——摘要

条目3a:引言——这个案例有什么独特之处,它对科学文献有什么贡献?
条目3b:主要症状和/或重要的临床发现。
条目3c:主要诊断、治疗干预和结局。
条目3d:结论——该病例的主要收获是什么?

摘要与关键词、标题同样重要:关键词影响文章能否准确被同行检索到,标题影响同行决定是否阅读摘要,摘要影响同行决定是否阅读全文。

写好摘要既难也不难。难在于摘要是一篇文章的高度总结,需要作者对全文有全面深刻的理解,才能梳理出全文最重要的创新点是什么、对同行有什么价值,才能写好摘要。不难在于已有既成的框架,只要作者厘清脉络,想要写好也没有想象那么难。条目3a,简要交代研究的背景,并且通过对已有文献的理解进行对比,单刀直入点出这篇文章的创新和独特之处,一上来就抓住读者的注意力。然后,条目3b和3c涵盖了整个病例的主要信息,需要作者讲故事,即什么样的患者,有什么样的症状,做了什么治疗,最后结局如何。通过此文,作者认为最主要的关注点、临床发现是什么。最后,条目3d,作者在上述背景和结果发现的基础上,给出结论:这则病例对同行/这个领域到底有什么具体帮助和作用。

不良报告示范[6]:

Awareness of the immune-related adverse event of programmed cell death protein-1 (PD-1) inhibitor-induced pneumonitis is important. Herein, we report the clinical course of 3 patients suspected to have PD-1 inhibitor-induced pneumonitis after cessation of PD-1 inhibitor treatment. In case 1, a 62-year-old man was diagnosed with stag... he died 8 weeks after the onset of the pneumonitis. We report pneumonitis after discontinuation of ICIs in 3 patients. We confirm that, although uncommon, PD-1 inhibitor-induced irAEs can develop after treatment discontinuation. Further accumulation of cases and clarification of the clinical features of patients with irAEs, such as the time of onset, imaging findings, and treatment outcomes are needed.

解析：这篇病例系列文章在条目3b和3c方面报告得不错，详细讲述了每个患者的诊治经过，包括随访结局等。3d结论也有指示意义，即PD-1抑制药有关的免疫相关不良事件可能会在停药后发生，提醒同行留意。但作者没有点出来这则病例的创新点，第一句说了这个内容很重要，然后就没有下文了。如果要改，可以写成免疫抑制药相关不良事件绝大多数出现于用药期间，目前有关在停药后仍然出现不良事件的文献如何，而这篇文章在已有文献基础上，补充了什么，然后再介绍三则病例，这样自明性和吸引力都会提高。

欠佳报告示范[7]：

Indwelling urethral catheter placement is a common and comparatively safe procedure. Misplacement of a urethral catheter into the upper urinary tract is unusual, and only a few cases have been reported. We describe the case of a 43-year-old man who presented with oliguria and had a history of chemotherapy for known metastatic lung cancer. As he had no history of urological disease, urethral catheterization was expected to be uneventful. The catheter was unable to be pulled back to the bladder neck once the balloon was inflated, and the patient expressed discomfort. Subsequent computed tomography revealed that the tip of the catheter was placed in the middle of the right ureter. Unbeknownst to the physicians before urethral catheterization, the patient had severe lower urinary tract symptoms and urinary bladder dysfunction with hydronephrosis, likely due to chemotherapy. Based on the patient's symptoms and imaging results, we judged the possibility of severe ureteral injury to be low. The malpositioned catheter was removed uneventfully after complete balloon deflation and then reinserted properly. He was admitted to the medical department but died as a result of an exacerbation of the underlying disease unrelated to the incident. If urethral catheter placement seems abnormal, physicians should aspirate and irrigate to confirm correct positioning before balloon inflation; then, they should carefully pull the inflated balloon near the neck of the bladder while monitoring the patient's symptoms. Although urethral catheter placement is comparatively safe, physicians must keep in mind that patients who have undergone chemotherapy might be at a risk for this rare complication.

解析:这篇病例报告的故事讲得非常完整,既给出了患者年龄(43岁)等信息,也给了重要的病史信息(已知转移性肺癌,化疗史,无泌尿系统疾病史),还阐述了整个诊断(输尿管损伤)、干预(尿道导尿)和结局(死亡)全经过。文章结论也很明确,即接受过化疗的患者有可能容易出现尿道导管误置入上尿路的情况。但文章的独特点、创新点还可以写得更好。作者认为该文的独特点是报道尿道导管误置入上尿路的病例很罕见,即这是一则罕见病例。这确实是该文的一个点,但不是独特点。那么,这一例的出现,和其他罕见病例的出现,有何不同呢?其实,再追究深一步即可:既往这一情况本身就很罕见,而该病例进一步补充了这样的一个信息,即既往接受过化疗的患者容易出现尿道导管误置入上尿路这一罕见的情况。独特点在于"接受过化疗"。

良好报告示范[8]:

Chyle leakage after modified radical neck dissection is a rare condition that could be occasionally life-threatening if untreated. We report the first case of successful management of a thoracic duct injury using *Viscum album* extract (Helixor-M). A 54-year-old woman diagnosed with papillary thyroid cancer of the right lobe of the thyroid with metastasis to cervical lymph node levels II-VI, bilaterally, underwent total thyroidectomy and modified radical neck dissection. Three days postoperatively, the surgical team identified a thoracic duct injury due to drainage of chyle from the Jackson-Pratt drain inserted in the right side of the patient's neck. Various medical treatments (octreotide, withdrawal of enteral feeding, and total parenteral nutrition) and surgical treatments [lymphatic ligation of cervical lymph node level IV and negative pressure wound therapy (vacuum-assisted closure)] were performed, but the drainage persisted. *Viscum album* extract (Helixor-M) was then injected through the drain. The dose of *Viscum album* extract was increased while being cautious of its adverse effects, such as nausea, vomiting, erythema, induration at the injection site, and flu-like symptoms. The injection was effective in stopping the drainage and the patient's condition improved, without recurrence. The patient was discharged on the 64th postoperative day without any further complications. Our results suggest that treatment of thoracic duct injury after neck surgery with *Viscum album* extract (Helixor-M) may be a novel, less invasive alternative approach to treat cases resistant to standard treatments.

解析:条目3a背景清晰——改良根治性颈部切除术后的乳糜漏是一种罕见的情况,如果不加以治疗,有时可能危及患者生命。独特点清晰——是第一个使用Helixor–M成功处理胸导管损伤的病例。条目3b和3c故事完整——患者,

54岁，女性，甲状腺右叶乳头状癌并转移到双侧颈部淋巴结Ⅱ~Ⅳ级；干预经过为甲状腺全切除术和改良根治性颈部切除术后3天出现糜烂物引流导致胸腔管道损伤，进一步行药物治疗（给出了药物名称）和手术治疗（给出了具体的手术方式）；对于患者结局，详细报告了不良反应和病情改善情况，包括是否复发，也给了具体随访时间和随访情况。条目3d结论清楚表态——用黏液囊提取物Helixor-M可以治疗对标准治疗有抵抗的病例，是创伤较小的替代方案。

（四）CARE条目4——引言

引言需用1~2个段落总结为何该病例是独一无二的（可能要包括参考文献）。

虽然这个条目明确说了1~2个段落，但笔者觉得这一条定得有点过于死板，3~4段也是可以的——只要作者能在引言中基于已有文献说清楚为什么这则病例是独一无二的和重要的。前面摘要说了文章独一无二的点是什么（即论点），引言其实就如立题依据一样，要通过文献梳理来说服读者，为什么是独一无二的（即用论据来论证）。而最常见的引言撰写问题就是论据不充分，论证的逻辑链条断裂。下面我们通过案例来说明。

不良报告示范[9]：

Pulmonary infectious complications are common after lung resections mainly with the form of atelectatic lung collapse and pneumonia. Development of such complications may lead to increased length of stay, length of stay in intensive care unit as well as increased 30-day and 90-day mortality. The severity of these complications is influenced by many factors i.e., their extent and mechanism of development, patient vulnerability, the compensatory reserves and others.

Conservative treatment of these complications usually includes antibiotics, use of mycolytics for reduced secretion volume, aggressive physiotherapy etc. In some cases, more aggressive interventions may be needed i.e., non-invasive ventilation and direct airway suctioning (with bronchoscopy or a tracheostomy). There are, however, rare cases in which the collapse persists, despite all the aforementioned measures, leading to the need for improvisation in an effort to avoid further surgery, which in borderline patients can be detrimental.

We herein present the technique of continuous endobronchial suctioning in a patient who after a complicated redo thoracotomy for lung cancer developed refractory collapse of the remaining upper lobe. This technique may be proven invaluable in the treatment of such demanding cases wherever the usual conservative measures fail. This article is presented in accordance with the CARE reporting checklist (available at http://dx.doi.org/10.21037/atm-20-3839).

解析：该引言第一段主要介绍肺切除术后肺部感染并发症的背景，即临床表现、病死率、严重性。第二段则过渡到治疗，从保守治疗（抗生素、肌醇类药物、物理治疗）说到更积极的治疗（无创通气、气道抽吸），再到这些治疗都可能失败的现状。第三段则直接点出此文的目的是介绍连续支气管内吸痰技术，并强调通常的保守措施都会失败，所以这种技术非常有价值。

这则引言被认定为报告不佳就是因为作者在论证该病例独一无二的特点和重要性的过程中，论据不完整且逻辑链条断裂。以往有没有通过连续支气管内吸痰来处理肺切除术后肺部感染并发症的文献呢？作者没有说明，也就是论据缺失。那么，如果以往已有，与以往类似的也用连续支气管内吸痰来处理的病例相比，该病例的不同之处在哪里？如果既往没有，作者也应该清楚说明这个情况，并以此来论证其重要性。

良好报告示范[10]：

More than 90% of chronic renal failure patients develop secondary hyperparathyroidism (HPT). This is due to several factors: first is phosphate retention due to loss of nephrons function; second is vitamin D resistance by decreased responsiveness of the uremic intestine; and third is the inability of kidneys to hydroxylate 25-hydroxycholecalcifrol. These factors will predispose nodular hyperplasia due to the prolonged stimulation of parathyroid cell growth due to high phosphate, low calcitriol, and hypocalcemia. Over time, and after the initiation of hemodialysis, persistent parathyroid hyperfunction will result in the development of a tertiary HPT from the secondary hyperplasia. The development of multiple parathyroid adenomas in a patient with tertiary HPT who is on hemodialysis is rare. There is only one report case in Japan in 1982 of a known tertiary HPT patient on hemodialysis with a parathyroid adenoma. A similar case of a Secondary HPT with an adenoma was reported in 2014. To the best of our knowledge, this case was the first to be described as "true" tertiary HPT with multiple parathyroid adenomas, secondary hyperplasia of the remaining two parathyroid glands and a PTH level reaching 4,267.2 pg/mL. For clearness, we present this case following the CARE reporting checklist (available at http://dx.doi.org/10.21037/acr-20-115).

解析：这则引言详细地引用了以往类似病例并与之作比较，即1982年报告的三级继发性甲状旁腺功能亢进患者在血液透析中出现甲状旁腺瘤，2014年报告的一例类似的二级继发性甲状旁腺功能亢进伴甲状旁腺腺瘤，而本病例是第一个被描述为真正的三级继发性甲状旁腺功能亢进且有多个甲状旁腺腺瘤的病例。

良好报告示范[11]：

Anterior lumbar interbody fusion (ALIF) is a commonly performed procedure for lumbar degenerative disease with excellent results, particularly for discogenic low back pain. However, reported complications associated with ALIF include vessel injury, retrograde ejaculation, and ureteral and viscus organ injury. The development of a varicocele after ALIF has not been previously described in the literature. We report a case of varicocele as a complication of ALIF. We describe the occurrence of a varicocele following ALIF, its possible pathophysiology and treatment options. We present the following case in accordance with the CARE reporting checklist (available at http://dx.doi.org/10.21037/jss-20-609).

解析：这则引言非常言简意赅，指出独一无二的点就是报告了腰椎前路椎体间融合术的并发症。以往文献都只涉及血管损伤、逆行射精、输尿管和内脏器官损伤，没有报告术后出现精索静脉曲张这一并发症的情况。而这则病例报告了这一并发症，并提供了可能的病理生理和治疗方案。

（五）CARE条目5——患者信息

条目5a：去除患者身份的具体信息。
条目5b：主诉和症状。
条目5c：医疗、家庭和社会心理史，包括相关的遗传信息。
条目5d：过去的相关干预措施及结果。

患者信息这个大条目的4个子条目中，最常见的报告不当有：只是简单地把患者姓名匿名化却仍然报告了很多不必要的可能泄露患者身份的信息，漏掉重要的既往史，漏掉重要的既往干预。

什么样的患者信息算泄露个人身份，什么样的不算呢？总的原则是，尽量减少患者的个人信息中和病例病情无关的信息。披露年龄、性别、国籍等通常没有问题，而对于患者的居住地、职业、个人喜好等，只有当与病例有关时才能披露。比如，一位患者职业是矿工，如果这个病例是一个尘肺病病例，那就必须交代这个职业；但如果这个病例是一个糖尿病病例，那就没有必要报告其职业。再比如，如果一个患者因为剧烈运动而受伤就诊，受伤和运动强度有关，而这个患者正好是职业运动员，就应该报告职业；相反，如果这个患者患的是其他疾病，如肺癌，那就没有必要报告职业。

良好报告示范[12]：

A 35-year-old high-level endurance female athlete (weight 59 kg, height 168 cm; BMI 20.9 kg/m^2; resting blood pressure 105/57 mmHg; resting heart rate 66 bpm) attended the clinic complaining about chest pain and dyspnea on exertion, dizziness and presyncope occurring during maximum-intensity exercise training sessions. She had been performing 15 hours/week of exercise endurance training for 20 years until symptoms' presentation. No history of cardiovascular disease, cardiovascular risk factors and no medical-surgical history of interest were reported. She denied the use of doping and/or stimulants, particularly caffeine. She had never smoked and other risk factors such as diabetes and hypertension were ruled out. No family history of sudden death, syncope, or known cardiac disease was reported.

解析：这则引言没有泄露任何涉及个人隐私的信息，且关键个人信息报告到位，包括年龄、性别、BMI、血压、心率、与病情相关的职业——高水平耐力的运动员。主诉和症状：进行最大强度运动训练时出现胸痛，用力时呼吸困难、头晕、晕厥，出现症状前已进行15小时/周的耐力训练20年。相关个人史和既往干预：没有心血管疾病史和心血管危险因素，没有相关的内外科病史，否认使用过兴奋药和/或刺激物，从未吸烟，并排除了其他危险因素，如糖尿病和高血压，没有猝死、晕厥或已知心脏疾病的家族史报告。

（六）CARE条目6——临床发现

临床发现中需描述重要的检查和重要的临床发现。

条目6的报告质量大都很好，很少看到报告不佳的情况，详细报告患者做了哪些检查，通过这些检查有什么重要的发现即可。考虑到篇幅，不再做案例介绍，读者可在第四章的案例中查看细节。

（七）CARE条目7——时间轴

以时间轴的形式组织诊治照护信息，包括历史信息和当前信息。

条目7的报告非常不佳，所以笔者将重点介绍。笔者审核过的病例中，要么是作者错误理解时间轴，要么是绘制的时间轴没有传达核心信息。衡量一份时间轴是否优秀的标准是判断其是否可以独立成文，即通过时间轴（图或表），在不看全文时便可知悉该病例传达的最主要的信息。

不良报告示范[13-14]:

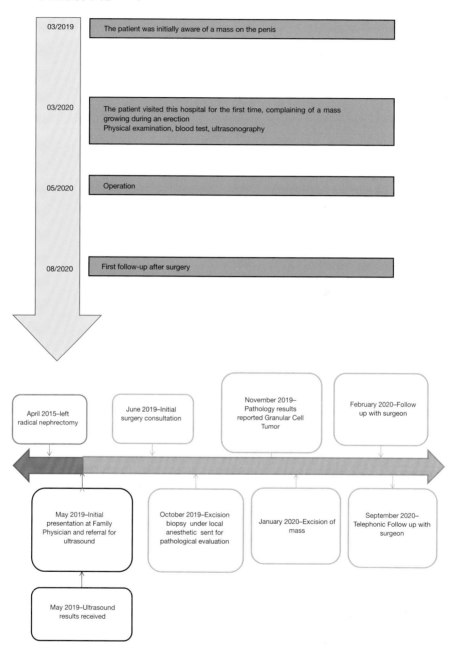

解析：这两份时间轴都给了详细的时间，但是核心信息大量缺失，更像是一份"流水账"。比如写了2020年5月做了手术，但没有提及做了什么手术，

手术结果如何；写了2020年8月做了术后第一次随访，但没有说明随访情况。不能只是呈现做了什么，还要给出做了这些后效果究竟如何。

不良报告示范[15]：

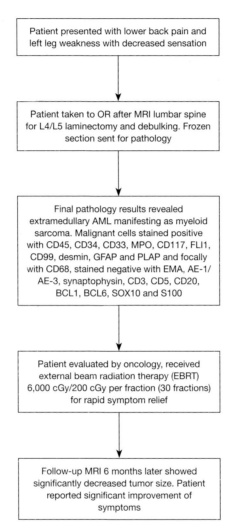

解析：这一份时间轴把想要表达的核心信息都写出来了。但没有体现"时间"，且文字过多，使读者阅读体验不佳，便利程度也与看全文的详细描述相近。

良好报告示范[16]：

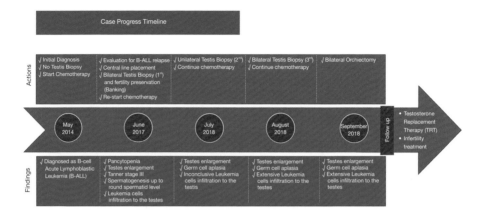

解析：这一份时间轴不仅把关键信息都囊括了，而且时间线非常清晰。值得借鉴的是，这个案例中，作者把做了什么和发现了什么分开呈现，阅读起来信息很清楚，而且随访也没有遗漏。

良好报告示范[17]：

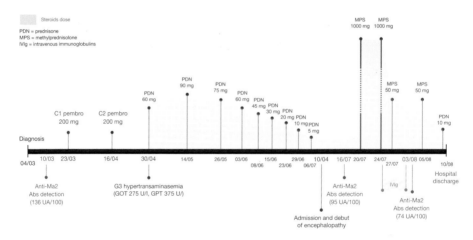

解析：这份时间轴的优点与上一例时间轴一样，此外，这一份时间轴可供借鉴的还有药物剂量的可视化呈现。由于该病例核心信息是PDN和MPS用药剂量的调整，所以作者重点突出了这个点，给了所有药物的剂量，并用绿点的高低来呈现用药剂量的大小，非常直观。

良好报告示范[18]：

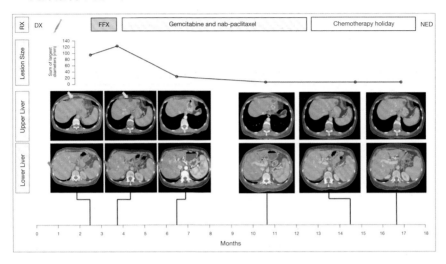

解析：可以看到，这是一份信息密度很大的时间轴。在这张图中，既有整个0~18个月时间的呈现，也有治疗方案的呈现，还有影像学的改变情况。值得借鉴的是，作者直接用可视化的方式把病灶大小动态呈现了出来，读者读起来十分清楚直观，一下子就可以抓住在每个治疗方案之后病灶大小的变化情况。如果作者能用具体的年和月来表现时间会更好，因为疾病的诊治是有时代背景的，直接写明何年何月比第几天、几个月更加有自明性。

良好报告示范[19]：

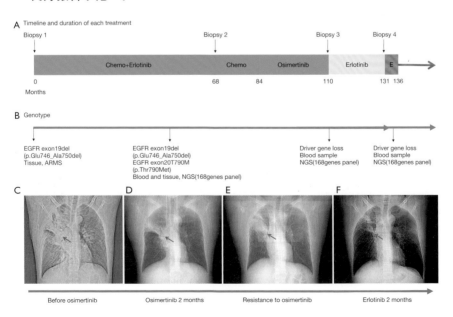

解析：这份时间轴除了有上述提及的优点外，还根据想要表达的不同信息分成了A、B、C三个模块，用时间轴进行对应串接。从这份时间轴中，能看到这个患者一开始的影像学表现、EGFR基因型、整个治疗经过和在哪几个时间点又做了基因检测，整个过程中的基因型变化和影像学变化也清楚明了。如果这份时间轴能再加上患者之后的随访情况会更完善。

（八）CARE条目8——诊断评估

条目8a：诊断检查，如体格检查、实验室检查、影像、调查。

条目8b：诊断方面的挑战，如是否有条件开展检查、费用或文化挑战。

条目8c：诊断，包括鉴别诊断。

条目8d：预后，如肿瘤学中的分期（如适用）。

与条目6一样，条目8的报告质量总体很好。主要是客观陈述对患者做了什么检查，发现了什么，诊断经过等。所以，囿于篇幅，也不再过多说明，读者可通过第四章的案例详细了解。

（九）CARE条目9——治疗干预

条目9a：治疗干预的类型，如药物、手术、预防、自我护理等。

条目9b：治疗干预的管理，如剂量、强度、持续时间。

条目9c：治疗干预的变化，需要提供改变理由。

条目9的报告，需要改善的地方主要有两点：一是作者常给出大致的干预情况而没有交代具体管理，比如没有给出剂量、强度、持续时间等；二是对治疗方案的更改，没有给出原因，让人担忧更改的合理性。

良好报告示范[19]：

Platinum-based chemotherapy, comprising of docetaxel plus cisplatin, was administered for two cycles. Subsequently, treatment was changed to erlotinib (150 mg per day, orally) as maintenance therapy and achieved partial response. The patient maintained a partial response for 5 years and 6 months. CT evaluation indicated an increase in lung mass size, indicating that the patient had progressive disease. Treatment was changed to a combination of pemetrexed plus endostar, with partial response for 16 months. Disease progression was evaluated after new metastatic lesions were detected in the lung. Blood and tissue samples were both sent for NGS using a panel consisting of 168 genes (LungPlasma, Burning Rock Biotech, Guangzhou, China), which revealed EGFR T790M in the tumor (Figure 1C). Treatment was then changed to osimertinib (80 mg per day, orally) and the patient achieved partial response for 26 months (Figure 1D), before disease progression, indicated by the discovery of new lung metastases (Figure 1E). Targeted sequencing of blood and tissue samples using the same 168-gene panel revealed the disappearance of both EGFR exon 19del and T790M. No other actionable mutations were detected.

解析：这份报告详细给出了各治疗的具体药物名称、剂量、间隔等，并且陈述了治疗方案的更换原因，即疾病进展了。

（十）CARE条目10——随访和结局

条目10a：临床医生和患者评估的结果（如果有）。
条目10b：重要的后续诊断和其他测试结果。
条目10c：干预的依从性和耐受性，以及如何评估的。
条目10d：不良和预期之外的事件。

条目10的报告不符合的情况并不罕见，要么是没有报告随访和结局，要么是报喜不报忧——没有任何关于不良反应的描述。这样一来，读者便不知道有没有随访、最后患者怎样了、这个方案到底安不安全，获得的信息是不完整的。

良好报告示范[19]：

Erlotinib was re-administered in March, 2017 and has achieved a partial response for 26 months and he continued to benefit from erlotinib as of this writing (Figure 1F, 2). The entire treatment time line and adverse events reported by the patient during the course of the treatment are summarized in Table S1.

Table S1 Summary of treatment regimen and adverse events observed from the patient

Treatment regimen	Treatment line	Progression-free Survival (months)	Adverse events
Docetaxel plus cisplatin + sub-erlotinib	1	68	Grade I rash
Pemetrexed plus endostar	2	16	None
Osimertinib	3	26	Grade II rash and Grade I diarrhea
Erlotinib	4	26+	Grade I rash and Grade I diarrhea

解析：作者一直随访到撰稿时间点为止，给出了随访结局即partial response，并且用表格详细汇总了不良反应和对应的无疾病进展期。

（十一）CARE条目11——讨论

条目11a：对本病例报告的优点和局限性进行科学讨论。
条目11b：引用参考文献以展开对相关医学文献的讨论。
条目11c：给出结论的科学依据，包括对可能原因的评估。
条目11d：用一个无参考文献的段落来给出结论，说明本病例报告的主要启示。

条目11最常见的问题就是作者不写局限性。一些作者写了局限性，但经常回避要害，只谈及一些皮毛的不足或只提及所有病例报告难以避免的回顾性和样本量问题，而没有涉及实质内容层面的讨论。

欠佳报告示范[20]：

There are methodological limitations, as like most of the case reports, in terms of the retrospective nature of the report and the fact that it lacks the power for generalization.

解析：这份报告只谈及研究是回顾性的以及单个病例外推性不足的问题，说得都合理，但没有阐述内容层面。

良好报告示范[21]：

A limitation of this study is that plasma concentrations of rosuvastatin and its metabolites were not measured. However, the adherence of the patient to the prescribed treatment was ensured using a validated adherence questionnaire and regular follow-up calls.

解析：谈及了最核心的局限性——没有测量罗苏伐他汀及其代谢物的血浆浓度。

良好报告示范[22]：

Our study found a very rare CFHR3-CFHR1 copy number gain as the cause of atypical HUS. However, our study has some limitations. First, a functional study was not performed on the discovered mutations. In addition, the mechanism of how CFHR3-CFHR1 copy number gain generated atypical HUS could not be revealed. Second, although no family member with similar symptoms was found, it is a limitation of our study that genetic testing of the family members was not performed because of that.

解析：这份报告客观报告了几个主要的局限性——没有对发现的突变体进行功能研究，机制不清，也没有对家族成员进行基因检测。

良好报告示范[23]：

A potential limitation of this case series is the lack of long-term follow-up data for the first patient who showed evidence of progression of NSCLC on first surveillance imaging after starting lorlatinib. While many severe cases of DI-ILD occur acutely, reports of long-term safety data will be important in the future to assess the potential for delayed adverse events secondary to lorlatinib.

解析：这份报告的局限性是缺乏第一个患者的长期随访数据。

即便笔者将上述三个案例划作"良好报告示范"类别，这几个案例也并非完美。在局限性的基础上，再给出这些局限性可能给结果、结论带来的影响和不确定性会更好。另外，还可以给出解决这些局限性的具体方案。

（十二）*CARE*条目12——患者观点

患者观点，即用1~2个段落分享患者对所接受治疗的看法。

条目12主要想体现患者维度的看法，一来可以避免医务工作者过度乐观地报告，二来可以体现患者真正关心的点。在大多数情况下很难获得这条，比如患者出院后联系不上，但是能报告是最好的。

良好报告示范[21]：

I have had high cholesterol since I was a child and it has been an issue because of the delayed response to treatments and of many adverse reactions to medications, especially simvastatin. The authors have been very attentive towards me throughout the whole study and discovered possible variants that may delay my response to rosuvastatin and influence the pain that I have felt when using statins. I am very happy for knowing the cause of my problem and I would like to thank the authors for this possible diagnosis. This has improved my perspectives of cholesterol treatment.

解析：这则案例的患者观点很好地体现了患者尤其感谢医者是因为医者关注到他对罗苏伐他汀反应延迟的情况。整个治疗过程使得患者对胆固醇治疗的看法得到了很大改善。

良好报告示范[24]：

Our patient reported the following about his experience: "Throughout the process of my clinical care, I was informed about the concerns, doubts and problems that raised the diagnosis and treatment of my disease. I was aware of the risks of the surgical procedure, especially of facial nerve damage. Although during the first postoperative months I was concerned about the difficulty in moving my facial muscles, over time I have recovered normal facial mobility. Currently I can do my usual activity without any problem. However, I perceive a slight hollow in the preauricular area, but I am happy with the result obtained."

解析：这则案例的患者观点体现了患者的担心点——术后面部肌肉运动，患者认为仍然有待改进的地方——耳前区有轻微的凹陷，以及患者对治疗总体感受——满意。

（十三）*CARE*条目13——知情同意

患者是否知情同意？如有需要，请提供知情同意书。

根据期刊要求，作者可能需要尽可能在发表该病例前取得患者知情同意。患者有权决定作者能否将该病例以文章的方式进行发表而在全世界范围传播。

如果有些情况下无法取得患者知情同意，比如患者离世，作者也需要向编辑部说明情况。

报告示范[15]：

A written informed consent was obtained from the patient. Kern Medical Institutional Review Board granted ethical approval to report this case (Study # 20029).

报告示范[25]：

The patient gave his written informed consent for his personal and clinical details along with any identifying images to be published in this study.

报告示范[17]：

Written informed consent was obtained from the patient for the publication of this case report.

解析：以上几个案例值得借鉴的点是都清楚告知获得了患者的知情同意，一是给出了伦理审批信息和审批号；二是详细解释患者同意公布其个人和临床细节以及图像；三是明确说明患者同意发表其病例。

三、未来之路：如何更大范围提高病例报告的报告质量？

前文用了大量篇幅来详细剖析CARE的每个条目，以期获得读者对CARE条目更深刻的理解。但与此同时也应该看到，病例报告质量仍然欠佳的现状背后，还有许多其他原因。那么，有多大程度是因为期刊没有采纳CARE？有多大程度是因为期刊空喊口号，敷衍执行？又有多大程度是因为CARE本身存在问题？

就期刊采纳而言，如第一章所述，CARE官网显示，明确采纳CARE的有逾120本期刊，这一数据还没有包括AME出版社旗下60多本期刊以及其他类似AME的情况。我们可以由此估计，当前明确采纳CARE的期刊在200本左右，也可能更多。如第一章所述，仅2020年发表病例报告的期刊便逾3 600种。这样一看，这200本也只占不到6%。令人欣慰的是，越来越多的期刊加入采纳CARE这个队伍中来，这是一个很好的趋势。

就期刊执行而言，显然还有更大发力空间。虽然如*JAMA*、*BMJ Case Reports*、*Clinical Case Reports*以及AME出版社旗下60多本期刊都已明确强制要求作者按CARE来报告病例，但仍然不够。

就CARE本身而言，其的确并不完美。首先，其十分强调独一无二的点，而对一些虽不够独特，但同样经典及很有教育意义的病例不够重视。其次，截至笔者撰稿，自其发布以来，已有8年未更新。再者，其对药物治疗领域更为重视，而对手术领域的覆盖度不够。最后，它没有具体说明病例系列的文章应该怎么报告。

　　总之，改善病例报告的报告质量绝非单靠制定者制定出CARE、期刊采纳CARE、期刊执行CARE、作者按CARE报告病例中的任何一环就能实现。病例报告的报告质量需要指南制定者、期刊编辑、同行评议人员、作者和读者等多方的共同努力。很高兴，至少，CARE已为我们迈出了提高病例报告的报告质量的第一步。并且，期刊编辑、同行评议人员、作者也都取得了长足进步。未来，希望我们能广泛地推荐它，更好地使用它，并继续完善它。

参考文献

[1]　Seguel-Moraga P，Onetto JE，E Uribe S. Reporting quality of case reports about dental trauma published in international journals 2008-2018 assessed by CARE guidelines[J]. Dent Traumatol，2021，37(2)：345-353.

[2]　Park JH，Lee S，Kim TH，et al. Current status of case reports and case series reported by Korean Medicine doctors in primary clinics：A systematic review[J]. Integr Med Res，2020，9(4)：100417.

[3]　De Vito A，Taranath A，Dahmoush H，et al. Neuroimaging manifestations of epidermal nevus syndrome[J]. Quant Imaging Med Surg，2021，11(1)：415-422.

[4]　Zivkovic I，Milacic P，Mihajlovic V，et al. Surgical treatment of ascending aorta floating thrombus in a patient with recent SARS-CoV-2 infection[J]. Cardiovasc Diagn Ther，2021，11(2)：467-471.

[5]　Schiopu SRI，Käsmann L，Schönermarck U，et al. Pembrolizumab-induced myocarditis in a patient with malignant mesothelioma：plasma exchange as a successful emerging therapy-case report[J]. Transl Lung Cancer Res，2021，10(2)：1039-1046.

[6]　Kimura H，Sone T，Araya T，et al. Late-onset programmed cell death protein-1 inhibitor-induced pneumonitis after cessation of nivolumab or pembrolizumab in patients with advanced non-small cell lung cancer：a case series[J]. Transl Lung Cancer Res，2021，10(3)：1576-1581.

[7]　Cho SK，Kim MS，Chung HS，et al. Transurethral Foley catheter misplacement into the upper urinary tract in a patient with a history of lung cancer and chemotherapy：a case report and considerations to keep in mind[J]. Transl Androl Urol，2021，10(3)：1347-1351.

[8]　Kim CW，Kim JS，Lee AH，et al. Viscum album extract (Helixor-M) treatment for thoracic duct injury after modified radical neck dissection：a case report[J]. Gland Surg，2021，10(2)：832-836.

[9]　Kouritas V，Ross N，Bilyy A，et al. Continuous endobronchial suctioning for refractory post lobectomy lung atelectasis：a case report[J]. Ann Transl Med，2021，9(9)：815.

[10]　Assiri SA，Khurshid A，Thawabeh A. Two parathyroid adenomas in a Saudi female on

hemodialysis diagnosed with tertiary hyperparathyroidism: a case report[J]. AME Case Rep, 2021, 5: 4.

[11] Okamon DJM, Chenin L, Bocco A, et al. Varicocele complicating an anterior lumbar interbody fusion: a case report[J]. J Spine Surg, 2021, 7(1): 114-117.

[12] de la Guía-Galipienso F, Sanchis-Gomar F, Quesada-Dorador A. Diagnostic electrophysiological study in a highly trained young woman with presyncopal symptoms during exercise: a case report[J]. Ann Transl Med, 2021, 9(2): 177.

[13] Kim SH, Ahn H, Kim KH, et al. Penile schwannoma mistaken for hemangioma: a rare case report and literature review[J]. Transl Androl Urol, 2021, 10(6): 2512-2520.

[14] Rehan S, Paracha H, Masood R, et al. Granular cell tumor of the abdominal wall, a case report and review of literature[J]. AME Case Rep, 2021, 5: 28.

[15] Bhandohal JS, Moosavi L, Garcia-Pacheco I, et al. Isolated myeloid sarcoma of lumbar spine without bone marrow involvement: a rare case report and treatment dilemma[J]. AME Case Rep, 2021, 5: 27.

[16] Abdelaal O, Deebel NA, Zarandi NP, et al. Fertility preservation for pediatric male cancer patients: illustrating contemporary and future options; a case report[J]. Transl Androl Urol, 2021, 10(1): 520-526.

[17] Albarrán V, Pozas J, Rodríguez F, et al. Acute anti-Ma2 paraneoplastic encephalitis associated to pembrolizumab: a case report and review of literature[J]. Transl Lung Cancer Res, 2021, 10(7): 3303-3311.

[18] King DA, Rahalkar S, Bingham DB, et al. Pancreatic INI1-deficient undifferentiated rhabdoid carcinoma achieves complete clinical response on gemcitabine and nab-paclitaxel following immediate progression on FOLFIRINOX: a case report[J]. J Gastrointest Oncol, 2021, 12(2): 874-879.

[19] Liu L, Lizaso A, Mao X, et al. Rechallenge with erlotinib in osimertinib-resistant lung adenocarcinoma mediated by driver gene loss: a case report[J]. Transl Lung Cancer Res, 2020, 9(1): 144-147.

[20] Mak SKD, Chan NCD, Nolan CP, et al. Post-op lumbar subdural hygroma: a case report[J]. J Spine Surg, 2021, 7(2): 244-248.

[21] Dagli-Hernandez C, de Freitas RCC, Marçal EDSR, et al. Late response to rosuvastatin and statin-related myalgia due to SLCO1B1, SLCO1B3, ABCB11, and CYP3A5 variants in a patient with Familial Hypercholesterolemia: a case report[J]. Ann Transl Med, 2021, 9(1): 76.

[22] Choi HS, Yun JW, Kim HJ, et al. Atypical hemolytic uremic syndrome after childbirth: a case report[J]. Ann Transl Med, 2021, 9(1): 79.

[23] Myall NJ, Lei AQ, Wakelee HA. Safety of lorlatinib following alectinib-induced pneumonitis in two patients with ALK-rearranged non-small cell lung cancer: a case series[J]. Transl Lung Cancer Res, 2021, 10(1): 487-495.

[24] Rollon-Mayordomo A, Avellaneda-Camarena A, Gutierrez-Domingo A, et al. Synchronous occurrence of IgG4-related sialadenitis and ductal carcinoma of the parotid gland: a case report[J]. Gland Surg, 2021, 10(6): 2069-2075.

[25]　Pous A, Izquierdo C, Cucurull M, et al. Immune-checkpoint inhibitors for lung cancer patients amid the COVID-19 pandemic: a case report of severe meningoencephalitis after switching to an extended-interval higher flat-dose nivolumab regimen[J]. Transl Lung Cancer Res, 2021, 10(4): 1917-1923.

*作者：*张开平，AME出版社
*校对：*林瑶，AME出版社
　　　杨芳慧，AME出版社
　　　尚炳含，AME出版社

第三章 "治疗"病例报告报告质量不佳：
《病例报告指南》使用说明书

在了解了CARE之于病例报告的重要性，以及知悉如何按CARE的13个条目撰写病例报告后，我们还要知道如何在日常工作中灵活运用CARE，以发挥其最大功效。

不同角色的人看待同一事物的观点和角度不尽相同。在病例报告的发文过程中，主要围绕着这三类人群：作者、同行评议人员、期刊编辑。当然，在特定情况下，这三种身份也能任意转换。如果我们把病例报告的报告不规范比作一种"疾病"，那CARE无疑就是这一"疾病"的一剂"良药"。在此，本文将提供一份病例报告"质量不佳"的"疾病"诊断书，并针对作者、同行评议人员和期刊编辑这三类人群提供如何有效使用CARE的"药品使用说明书"。欢迎大家对号入座！

病例报告质量不佳诊断书[1]					
患者姓名	病例报告	科室	临床各科室	日期	2013 年

检查部位：全身
主要病情：
患者常伴有报告不完整、不准确、不一致、不规范等症状，并具有一定的传染性。
- 报告不完整：常表现为患者关键信息、重要病史、治疗干预细节、随访、不良反应、不足之处等信息的缺失。
- 报告不准确：常表现为措辞含糊，如无明确时间、地点，只交代药品种而无药物名称、剂量、疗程，无具体随访时长等情况。
- 报告不一致：常表现为前言不搭后语或信息前后矛盾。
- 报告不规范：常表现为未在标题和关键词中说明其病例报告的身份、使用药品商品名而非化学名／通用名、未取得患者知情同意等情况。
初步诊断：病例报告报告质量不佳
治疗建议：CARE（2013）[1]
　　　　　CARE 解释与说明性文件（2017）[2]

*CARE*使用说明书[1]

请仔细阅读说明书并在专业人士指导下使用

标准来源：EQUATOR Network[3] & *CARE*官网[1]

[药品名称]

通用名称：CARE（2013）

汉语拼音：CARE Zhinan（2013）

英文名称：CAse REport Guidelines（2013）

[药物组成] 本品包含一份清单、一份解释与说明性文件。

[作用类别] 本品为基于共识的临床病例报告指南。

[药理作用] 本品通过13个清单条目，对病例报告整体从标题至总结进行逐个指导，从而提高病例报告的报告质量。

[适应证] 病例报告"报告质量不佳"这一"疾病"。

[用法用量] 如下。

一、作者

（一）餐前服用（撰稿之前）

科学是站在巨人的肩膀上前进的。作者在动笔撰写稿件前需要大量阅读文献。由于在撰写文章前作者往往会参照已发表的病例报告，而病例报告"报告质量不佳"这一"疾病"的发病率又颇高，因此许多之后发表的病例报告极易被传染而患上"报告质量不佳"。

"报告质量不佳"的文献将严重影响我们评价其结果的可靠性。一旦不可靠的研究结果因"报告质量不佳"而变得"看起来""似乎"可靠，那么将产生更为深远的影响。对不可靠文献进行进一步深入研究，无异于在破损的地基上造楼，后续的一系列工作成果都随时可能在顷刻之间被摧毁。

因此，在动笔撰稿之前的阅读阶段，作者便可根据CARE对阅读的病例报告进行检查，通过评判其报告质量而批判性地理解其研究结果和结论。同时，参照CARE，可以让这个问题的答案更加明确：我手里的哪些病例可以用来撰写成病例报告以便跟同行交流？

（二）餐时服用（撰稿阶段）

虽然CARE制定的初衷是提高病例报告的报告质量，而并非被用作撰写模板，但CARE的13个条目的确是撰写病例报告的绝佳参考工具。

作者在动笔撰写病例报告时，完全可以将CARE打印出来，逐条核对，包括如何拟定标题、摘要中要展现哪些内容、引言如何布局、病例过程的描述顺序和关键信息、要讨论哪些点等。

这样做还可以将病例报告和临床病例记录明确地区分开来，并帮助作者厘清思路：这篇病例报告最大的创新/独特之处是什么？它最大的应用价值是什么？

（三）餐后服用（投稿阶段）

或许有人会说，诚然CARE清单对撰写病例报告具有很好的指导意义，但每个人书写风格不同，这可能会对成文的流畅性造成影响，因此拒绝在撰写阶段对照CARE。这当然可以，因为在下一阶段，CARE依旧可以发挥作用。

写完病例报告，进入投稿环节，这个过程从来都不容易：撰稿→投稿→被拒稿→改稿→重新投稿→再被拒稿→改稿→投稿→根据外审意见再改稿→接收。

这一过程不仅会消耗作者精力，还会对文章的时效性产生影响。同时，随着病例报告的不断发展，CARE始终占领着主要地位，期刊编辑要求作者在投稿时填写CARE清单逐渐成为一种趋势。更为重要的是，对于日夜翘首以盼收到修稿意见的作者而言，若是因为其文章报告不充分被同行评议人员质疑结果可信度而拒稿是件多么令人悔恨的事情。

鉴于此，作者完全可以在投稿时查看期刊投稿要求。对于清楚注明要求填写CARE清单的期刊，可以提前核对CARE清单：检查文章引言是否阐明清楚、报告患者信息是否遗漏既往病史、治疗干预情况是否交代详细等。这不仅是通过期刊编辑这道关卡的绝佳工具，也是让同行评议人员得以专业评估文章质量的重要前提。

二、同行评议人员

同行评议是学术成果发表过程中至关重要的一环，同行评议人员与作者以及期刊编辑之间存在着千丝万缕的联系。作为医学学术质量的"看门人"，同行评议人员在提高作者发表的病例报告质量、帮助期刊编辑作出合理公正的决策方面起关键作用[4]。

然而，没有天生具备同行评议能力的人。一位专业的同行评议人员的诞生，需要不断地积累审稿经验。CARE则可以助力这一积累过程：通过对照CARE清单，同行评议人员可以对病例报告的报告质量有更全面的了解。在此基础上，也方便进一步对其质量进行评估。而在日常的审稿过程中，通过检索开放获取期刊刊登的病例报告的相关资料（文章、开放的审稿意见、*CARE*清单），可以快速了解该病例报告并积累审稿方法[5-6]。

对于拥有丰富审稿经验的同行评议人员，*CARE*又有何用处呢？已有研究表明，与仅接受常规审稿意见的论文相比，那些额外接受基于*CARE*的审稿意见的论文总体质量更为上乘[7]。此外，在面对大量的审稿需求时，审稿质量和审稿效率缺一不可。*CARE*由经验丰富的各研究领域专家讨论后制定，确保重要信息完整报道。因此同行评议人员在拿到稿件后，可以根据*CARE*的Checklist对稿件报告的完整性进行初步审核，随后在框架符合要求的基础上对病例报告的内容进行审核。这在一定程度上也可以提高同行评议效率。

三、期刊编辑

作为同行评议过程的另一"看门人"，编辑还是整个出版流程（包括同行评议）的"看门人"。他们既需要遵循出版道德标准，遵循最佳编辑实践指南，也肩负着发表与全球健康息息相关的高质量研究这一社会责任[8]。

编辑长期与稿件为伍，接触各种类型的研究报告。相对于高质量系统评价和随机对照试验这些位于循证医学金字塔顶端的研究来说，病例报告似乎是最容易被忽视的存在。2003年，*Croatian Medical Journal*分析了影响因子（impact factor，IF）结构，发现病例报告的确是对IF贡献最小的一类研究（相对IF仅为0.19，而其他论著类报告为0.91，述评为0.63）[9]。这很容易让一些期刊编辑更青睐可带来更高引用率的文章类型。作为期刊编辑，首先便需要认识到病例报告的重要性。例如，一例例新型冠状病毒肺炎的病例报告，可能在帮助我们逐步了解这个疾病、了解有效的防控措施等方面发挥关键、及时的作用。

作为期刊编辑，还要重视*CARE*并严格按照*CARE*对病例报告的报告质量进行约束。虽然对*CARE*遵循情况的分析结果显示其依从性较差，但不少研究仍表明了*CARE*的有效性[10-13]。

首先，我们鼓励期刊编辑在日常工作中使用*CARE*规范病例报告；其次，我们也鼓励期刊编辑要求作者在文中引用*CARE*，以扩大其影响力；最后，我们鼓励期刊编辑在各学术研讨会中，不吝分享*CARE*对于病例报告发表的重要性。

四、紧密协作

无论是作者、同行评议人员还是期刊编辑，都应当认识到，想要用*CARE*"治"好病例报告"报告质量不佳"这一"疾病"，缺乏协作是行不通的，只有多方有效协作才能最大程度改善这一"疾病"：作者在动笔前便思虑清楚，动笔时章法明了，动笔后与期刊融洽对接；期刊编辑在收到稿件后详细审阅，提出具体建议，并将CARE清单和具体建议一并发送给同行评议人员；同行评议人员评估文章不仅要考虑文章学术质量，也要考虑文章的报告质量。

在此，我们呼吁作者遵循CARE，鼓励期刊编辑使用CARE，建议同行评议人员参考CARE审核文章报告质量。如此三方协作，切实提高病例报告的报告质量。

[注意事项]

1. 使用本品时，请严格依从给药疗程和用药方式使用，随意停药将影响本品疗效并导致病情反弹。研究[14]发现，如使用CARE后未发现病情改善（报告质量提高），可能与"服药"依从性差有关。

2. 本品仅用于提高病例报告的报告质量，不适用于直接评价病例报告学术质量。

[不良反应]

使用本品后的作者可能会因专注于完善稿件而出现疲乏、腰酸、背疼、"鼠标手"和情绪不佳等情况，可通过休息、调整心情等予以缓解。

[药物相互作用]

病例报告有时会以"病例报告及文献综述"的形式出现，可能需要"服用"包括CARE在内的两种报告指南。联用涉及到相互作用，具体可咨询期刊编辑或参见作者须知。

[贮藏条件]

开放获取：EQUATOR 协作网官网（https://www.equator-network.org/reporting-guidelines/care/）；CARE官网（https://www.care-statement.org/）。

[生产时间] 2021年9月

[有效期] CARE更新版发表前

[生产单位] AME出版社学术发展部

如有问题，请与生产商直接联系：academiceditor@amegroups.com

参考文献

[1] Gagnier JJ, Kienle G, Altman DG, et al. The CARE guidelines: consensus-based clinical case reporting guideline development[J]. Headache, 2013, 53(10): 1541-1547.

[2] Riley DS, Barber MS, Kienle GS, et al. CARE guidelines for case reports: explanation and elaboration document[J]. J Clin Epidemiol, 2017, 89: 218-235.

[3] Simera I, Altman DG, Moher D, et al. Guidelines for reporting health research: the

EQUATOR network's survey of guideline authors[J]. PLoS Med, 2008, 5(6): e139.

[4] Relman AS. Peer review in scientific journals—what good is it?[J]. West J Med, 1990, 153(5): 520-522.

[5] van Rooyen S, Godlee F, Evans S, et al. Effect of open peer review on quality of reviews and on reviewers' recommendations: a randomised trial[J]. BMJ, 1999, 318(7175): 23-27.

[6] Wicherts JM. Peer Review Quality and Transparency of the Peer-Review Process in Open Access and Subscription Journals[J]. PLoS One, 2016, 11(1): e0147913.

[7] Cobo E, Cortés J, Ribera JM, et al. Effect of using reporting guidelines during peer review on quality of final manuscripts submitted to a biomedical journal: masked randomised trial[J]. BMJ, 2011, 343: d6783.

[8] Hames I. Peer Review and Manuscript Management in Scientific Journals: Guidelines for Good Practice[M]. Oxford: Blackwell Publishing, 2008.

[9] Kovacic N. Structure of the 2003 impact factor for Croatian medical journal[J]. Croat Med J, 2004, 45(6): 671-673.

[10] Calvache JA, Vera-Montoya M, Ordoñez D, et al. Completeness of reporting of case reports in high-impact medical journals[J]. Eur J Clin Invest, 2020, 50(4): e13215.

[11] Kim J, Eom YJ, Lee YS, et al. The Current Status of Quality of Reporting in Acupuncture Treatment Case Reports: An Analysis of the Core Journal in Korea[J]. Evid Based Complement Alternat Med, 2017, 2017: 5810372.

[12] Eldawlatly A, Alsultan D, Al Dammas F, et al. Adaptation of CARE (CAse REport) guidelines on published case reports in the Saudi Journal of Anesthesia[J]. Saudi J Anaesth, 2018, 12(3): 446-449.

[13] Schmelz B, Elsner P. [Quality of dermatological case reports in German-speaking journals: The Case Reporting (CARE) Guideline][J]. Hautarzt, 2018, 69(7): 602-605.

[14] Seguel-Moraga P, Onetto JE, E Uribe S. Reporting quality of case reports about dental trauma published in international journals 2008-2018 assessed by CARE guidelines[J]. Dent Traumatol, 2021, 37(2): 345-353.

作者：林瑶，AME出版社
审核修订：张开平，AME出版社
校对：杨芳慧，AME出版社
　　　尚炳含，AME出版社

第四章　病例报告示例

第一篇病例报告案例解析

Case Report

条目1

Dynamic changes of acquired T790M mutation and small cell lung cancer transformation in a patient with EGFR-mutant adenocarcinoma after first- and third-generation EGFR-TKIs: a case report

Shuxiang Ma, Zhen He, Hongyong Fu, Lili Wang, Xuan Wu, Zhe Zhang, Qiming Wang

Department of Internal Medicine, Henan Cancer Hospital, Affiliated Cancer Hospital of Zhengzhou University, Zhengzhou 450008, China

Correspondence to: Qiming Wang. Department of Internal Medicine, Henan Cancer Hospital, Affiliated Cancer Hospital of Zhengzhou University, 127 Dongming Road, Zhengzhou 450008, China. Email: qimingwang1006@126.com.

条目3a

条目3b、3c

条目3d

Abstract: Epithelial growth factor receptor (EGFR) T790M mutation and small cell lung cancer (SCLC) transformation are well-known resistance mechanisms acquired during treatment with EGFR tyrosine kinase inhibitors (TKIs). Various mechanisms sometimes coexist in patients. Here, we report a 57-year-old female diagnosed with stage IV lung adenocarcinoma, who harbored an EGFR exon 19 deletion mutation. This patient initially received gefitinib and progressed after 14 months. A repeat biopsy was performed, and the original EGFR exon 19 deletion and acquired exon 20 T790M mutation were identified. Then, pemetrexed plus carboplatin was administered as second-line and osimertinib as third-line treatment. Rapid progression and mixed response were observed after 2 months on osimertinib, with stable disease of the primary lung lesion but rapid growth of a right lower chest mass. The progressive chest lesion underwent biopsy, and the SCLC transformation was revealed. Furthermore, the patient was treated with etoposide and cisplatin, and she achieved disease control for 4 months. A fourth biopsy both for the primary lung lesion and the chest mass were finally conducted. Interestingly, the histopathology of the two different lesions showed adenocarcinoma and SCLC, respectively. The patient then rapidly suffered brain metastasis, and no EGFR mutations were detected in her cerebrospinal fluid (CSF). Overall survival (OS) of the patient was 29 months. This patient experienced concomitant resistance mechanisms of T790M mutation and SCLC transformation, which might have resulted from intra-tumor heterogeneity and drug-induced selection. Ultimately, this case reminds us that repeat biopsies are essential for patients receiving EGFR-TKIs in order to make appropriate treatment decisions according to the diverse mechanisms of acquired resistance.

Keywords: Case report; EGFR T790M mutation; osimertinib; small cell lung cancer (SCLC); transformation

条目2

Submitted Sep 30, 2019. Accepted for publication Jan 02, 2020.

doi: 10.21037/tlcr.2020.01.07

View this article at: http://dx.doi.org/10.21037/tlcr.2020.01.07

条目4

Introduction

Epidermal growth factor receptor (EGFR) inhibitors have revolutionized the treatment of EGFR-mutant non-small cell lung cancer (NSCLC) patients. Unfortunately, all patients will ultimately experience relapse with a median progression-free survival (PFS) of 7 to 16 months during the first- and second-generation EGFR-tyrosine kinase inhibitor (TKI) treatment (1,2). The major resistance mechanism is the EGFR T790M mutation within exon 20, observed in approximately 60% of resistant cases (3,4).

Osimertinib, a third-generation EGFR-TKI, is a pyrimidine-based irreversible inhibitor for both EGFR-activating mutations (e.g., exon 19 deletion or L858R) and T790M mutation. In AURA3, osimertinib was superior to

Transl Lung Cancer Res 2020;9(1):139-143 | http://dx.doi.org/10.21037/tlcr.2020.01.07

条目1：标题 写明最初的诊断或干预关注点，其后加上"case report"

报告到位。作者用PICOS方式拟定标题，并突出了最主要的点：P——EGFR突变的肺腺癌，I——第一代和第三代EGFR-TKIs，O——T790M突变和小细胞肺癌转化，S——病例报告。

条目2：关键词 2~5个点明该病例报告的诊断或干预的关键词，包括"case report"

关键词拟定到位。Keywords很好地体现出了标题中的PICOS原则，作者也没有遗漏case report。

条目3a：摘要 这个案例有什么独特之处，它对科学文献有什么贡献？

报告可以再改善，因为作者没有报告本病例的独特之处。作者已经在摘要中表示，EGFR T790M突变和小细胞肺癌转化是TKIs治疗期间耐药的机制。既然已经广为报告，为何读者还需要再读这篇文章？作者需要一针见血地指出此病例和以往病例的不同之处，让读者了解读了这篇病例报告会获得什么不一样的收获。

条目3b：摘要 主要症状和/或重要的临床发现
条目3c：摘要 主要诊断、治疗干预和结局

报告到位。作者完整报道了患者的主要信息：一名57岁的Ⅳ期肺腺癌女性，存在EGFR 19号外显子缺失突变；接受吉非替尼（第一代EGFR-TKI）治疗后，活检发现获得性20号外显子产生T790M突变，经过二线（培美曲塞联合卡铂）和三线（奥希替尼，第三代EGFR-TKI）治疗后，肺部病变稳定，但再次活检发现小细胞肺癌转化，并伴随脑转移。最后，报告了总生存期。

条目3d：摘要 结论——该病例的主要收获是什么？

报告到位，不是重复结果，而是根据结果得出经思考的经验总结。结论指出：对于接受EGFR-TKIs治疗的患者，重复活检必不可少，以便根据获得性耐药的不同机制作出适当的治疗决定。

条目4：引言 用1~2个段落总结为何该病例是独一无二的

作者很好地阐述了EGFR-TKI对EGFR突变的非小细胞肺癌患者的重要作用。奥希替尼作为第三代EGFR-TKI，对患者有良好的疗效，但患者也会产生耐药，转变为小细胞肺癌。作者没有指出该病例的独特性和价值，之前是否有过类似研究，这一点需要重点补充。

platinum plus pemetrexed in patients with T790M-positive NSCLC who progressed during prior EGFR-TKI therapy, achieving a median PFS of 10.1 months (5). However, similar to first- and second-generation EGFR-TKIs, resistance to osimertinib is inevitable. Numerous resistance mechanisms have been discovered to date, of which transformation to small cell lung cancer (SCLC) has been defined as a rare mechanism occurring in approximately 2% of patients (6,7).

Hence, we report a case in which T790M mutation and SCLC transformation appeared sequentially during treatment with first- and third-generation EGFR-TKIs. We present the following case in accordance with the CARE-Guideline (8).

Case presentation

条目5a、5b、5c

A 57-year-old never-smoking female complaining with intermittent cough presented in February 2015. Her father had been diagnosed with gastric adenocarcinoma and her sister with breast cancer. Physical examination suggested an Eastern Cooperative Oncology Group (ECOG) performance status of 1, and no significant abnormalities were found. Computed tomography (CT) scans of the chest showed a 20 mm × 14 mm mass in the middle lobe of the right lung, and two small nodules in the right middle lung, and right pleura (*Figure 1A*). Magnetic resonance imaging (MRI) of the brain and emission computed tomography (ECT) of the bone were also performed, and no other metastases were found. Both trans-bronchial biopsy and

条目6

Transl Lung Cancer Res 2020;9(1):139-143 | http://dx.doi.org/10.21037/tlcr.2020.01.07

条目5a：患者信息　去除患者身份的具体信息
条目5b：患者信息　主诉和症状
条目5c：患者信息　医疗、家庭和社会心理史，包括相关的遗传信息

作者报道了年龄、性别和吸烟史这些与疾病相关的信息，未泄露其他与病情无关的涉及患者身份的信息。主诉：间歇性咳嗽。家族史：父亲患有胃腺癌，姐姐患有乳腺癌。但作者未报道个人既往史，如果有会更好（条目5d）。

条目6：临床发现　描述重要的检查和重要的临床发现

报告到位。作者客观陈述了所有检查及重要发现，胸部CT显示右肺中叶有1个20 mm×14 mm的肿块，右中肺和右胸膜有2个小结节，其余检查结果正常。

条目7：时间轴　以时间轴的形式组织诊治照护信息，包括历史信息和当前信息

时间轴非常清晰，每个时间点对应的疾病进展和治疗都有清楚的标注，且

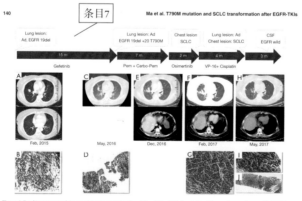

Figure 1 Graphic summary of the case. First biopsy at baseline of the right middle lung lesion (A) was adenocarcinoma with EGFR exon 19 deletion (B). The second biopsy of the enlarged primary lung lesion (C) after first-line gefitinib was adenocarcinoma with primary EGFR exon 19 deletion and acquired T790M mutation (D). After progression on second-line pemetrexed plus carboplatin, an enlarged primary lung lesion and new mass in the right lower chest were observed (E). The patient then took osimertinib as third-line treatment and rapid progression and mixed response were observed after 2 months (F). The progressive chest lesion underwent biopsy, and SCLC transformation was revealed (G). Etoposide plus cisplatin was administrated as fourth-line treatment yielding a response of partial response (H). A fourth biopsy for both the primary lung lesion and the chest mass was finally conducted. The histopathology of two different lesions showed SCLC (I) and adenocarcinoma (J), respectively. The magnification of pathologic graphs is 200×. EGFR, epithelial growth factor receptor; SCLC, small cell lung cancer.

注明了详细的年月，体现了治疗的时代背景。由于这则病例最重要的关注点，还有患者的T790M突变和小细胞肺癌转化，因此作者在时间轴中将这些关键信息和各阶段治疗对应起来。整个时间轴可以做到独立成文，在不读文章时也可知晓该病例的主要及重要概况。如果作者能在时间轴的前后增加疾病的既往史和随访结果，就完美了。

条目8a：诊断评估　诊断检查，如体格检查、实验室检查、影像、调查

报告到位。患者经支气管和胸膜病变活检，以及反转录聚合酶链式反应，诊断为伴有EGFR 19号外显子缺失突变的Ⅳ期肺腺癌。活检是诊断的"金标准"，诊断结果可靠。

条目9a：治疗干预　治疗干预的类型，如药物、手术、预防、自我护理等
条目9b：治疗干预　治疗干预的管理，如剂量、强度、持续时间

开始使用第一代EGFR-TKI，详细写明了药物的名称和剂量，如果作者能

Translational Lung Cancer Research, Vol 9, No 1 February 2020　　　141

条目8a

pleural lesion biopsy confirmed lung adenocarcinomas (*Figure 1B*). EGFR exon 19 deletion was identified via the reverse transcription-polymerase chain reaction (RT-PCR) method. So the diagnosis of this patient was stage IV lung adenocarcinoma with an EGFR exon 19 deletion mutation (cT3N0M1a according to TNM version 7).

条目9a、9b

Gefitinib (250 mg daily) was initiated as first-line treatment from March 2015, and the best response was partial response (PR) according to the Response Evaluation Criteria in Solid Tumor version 1.1 (RECIST 1.1). The disease progressed after 14 months, and repeat chest CT scans showed an enlarged right middle lobe mass (*Figure 1C*). Laboratory findings showed increased carcinoembryonic antigen (CEA) level of 11.1 ng/mL (normal range, 0 to 3.4 ng/mL) and neuron-specific enolase (NSE) of 15.44 ng/mL (normal range, 0 to 12.5 ng/mL) in the serum.

条目8d

A repeat biopsy of the right middle lung mass was performed and histologic analysis showed adenocarcinoma (*Figure 1D*). The results of immunohistochemistry (IHC) staining were positive for Napsin A, thyroid transcription factor-1 (TTF-1) and cytokeratin 7 (CK-7). Next-generation sequencing including 8 genes (EGFR, ALK, KRAS, ROS-1, BRAF, RET, ERBB2, MET) revealed original EGFR exon 19 deletion and acquired exon 20 T790M mutation.

条目9c

The third-generation EGFR-TKIs including osimertinib was not accessible in China until 2017, so pemetrexed

条目8d、9c①

(500 mg/m² intravenously on day 1, every 21 days) and carboplatin (AUC 5 intravenously on day 1, every 21 days) were administrated as second-line treatment. The patient achieved a response of PR and a PFS of 5 months. In October 2016, the chest CT scan showed an enlarged right middle lung mass (*Figure 1E*).

Then this patient was given osimertinib (80 mg daily) as third-line treatment. Regrettably, a mixed response was observed after 2 months, with stable disease of the lung lesions but a sharply increased right lower chest mass (*Figure 1F*). No metastases were found on brain MRI. The blood test showed significantly increases of NSE (from 24.9 ng/mL in December 2016 to 159.3 ng/mL in February 2017). Biopsy of the progressive chest lesion showed SCLC transformation (*Figure 1G*). The IHC staining results also showed a

条目8d、9c②

neuroendocrine morphology with CD56 and synaptophysin (SyN) positive, which was not seen in pre-osimertinib tumors, while Napsin A, TTF-1 and CK-7 were negative.

For fourth-line treatment, we chose etoposide (100 mg/m² intravenously on day 1 to 3) plus cisplatin (75 mg/m² intravenously on day 1, every 21 days), which is the standard

条目8d

regimen for advanced SCLCs. The level of NSE in serum was decreased dramatically to 14.97 ng/mL after two cycles of chemotherapy. The patient achieved a response of PR and a PFS of 4 months (*Figure 1H*). After progression, we did the fourth biopsy for the right middle lung mass and the chest mass. Interestingly, the chest mass showed SCLC (*Figure 1I*), while the histopathology of the lung mass showed adenocarcinoma (*Figure 1J*). This patient rapidly developed brain metastases in July 2017. No EGFR mutations were detected in her cerebrospinal fluid (CSF).

条目10b、10c、10d

The tolerability of this patient was well during treatment. No severe or unanticipated adverse events were reported. She died in September 2017, and the overall survival (OS) of this patient was 29 months.

Discussion

SCLC transformation is one of the resistance mechanisms associated with first-generation EGFR-TKIs, accounting for about 10% of all cases (7,9). Resistance to osimertinib is also inevitable and numerous mechanisms have been discovered to date. Acquired EGFR C797S mutation was thought to be the major mechanism (10). Meanwhile, SCLC transformation has also been reported as a rare resistance mechanism, accounting for about 2% of cases (6,7). Until now, fewer than 10 SCLC transformation cases after third-generation EGFR-TKIs have been reported in total (11-14). The durations from third-generation EGFR-TKI initiation to transformation is 6 to 18 months, which suggests that long-term exposure to TKI may be needed for SCLC transformation. Furthermore, genomic analysis has shown that the primary EGFR mutation can be universally maintained and the SCLC and EGFR T790M-positive clonal subpopulations seem to be distinct from each other (15).

条目11a

In our case, we report another metastatic adenocarcinoma patient harboring activating EGFR mutation who experienced T790M mutation and SCLC transformation dynamically after the treatment of first-generation EGFR-TKI gefitinib and third-generation EGFR-TKI osimertinib. Different from previously reported cases, the patient reported in our study experienced rapid SCLC transformation just 2 months after osimertinib initiation. Moreover, the case in our report lost T790M mutation as well as the primary EGFR exon 19 deletion after transformation, which might be a false test result because of the low sensitivity of CSF detection.

The mechanisms of SCLC transformation remain largely unresolved. Several studies have shown that

　　Transl Lung Cancer Res 2020;9(1):139-143 | http://dx.doi.org/10.21037/tlcr.2020.01.07

补充用法和用量会更好（如20 mg，每天3次）。

条目8d：诊断评估　预后，如肿瘤学中的分期（如适用）

对疾病进展的阐述清晰完整，包括CT扫描、血生化检查、右中肺肿块重复活检、免疫组织化学染色和基因测序的结果，疾病进一步进展，出现T790M突变。

条目9c：治疗干预　治疗干预的变化，需要提供改变理由

报告到位：提供了更改治疗方案的理由——疾病进展，并报告了具体治疗变化——患者改用培美曲塞联合卡铂的二线治疗（名称、剂量和用法描述较全面）。

条目8d：诊断评估　预后，如肿瘤学中的分期（如适用）
条目9c①：治疗干预　治疗干预的变化，需要提供改变理由

患者取得部分缓解和5个月无进展生存期，复查胸部CT显示右中肺肿块增大，疾病进展，再次更改治疗方案，使用奥希替尼（第三代EGFR-TKI）作为三线疗法。

条目8d：诊断评估　预后，如肿瘤学中的分期（如适用）
条目9c②：治疗干预　治疗干预的变化，需要提供改变理由

随后发现，肺部病变稳定，但右下胸肿块急剧增大，再次活检发现胸部肿块小细胞肺癌转化，血生化检查和免疫组织化学染色结果也有变化。因此，改用四线疗法治疗。

条目8d：诊断评估　预后，如肿瘤学中的分期（如适用）

血生化检查结果好转，患者再次取得部分缓解和4个月无进展生存期。后出现脑转移，脑脊液中没有发现EGFR突变。

条目10b：随访和结局　重要的后续诊断和其他测试结果
条目10c：随访和结局　干预的依从性和耐受性，以及如何评估的
条目10d：随访和结局　不良和预期之外的事件

报告到位：报告了患者对干预的耐受性（良好）和不良反应（未发生），以及随访结果（总生存期为29个月）。报告完整，做到了有始有终。

条目11a：讨论　对本病例报告的优点和局限性进行科学讨论

优点：作者提到第三代EGFR-TKI治疗后的小细胞肺癌转化病例总共不到10例，同时指出了本病例的创新点，即使用奥希替尼后仅2个月就经历了小细胞肺癌的快速转化，进一步丰富了原来的研究。这一点可以在摘要中简要提及以说明病例的独特之处。

局限性：谈到了本病例中不可控的局限性，即患者在小细胞肺癌转化后失去了T790M突变以及主要的EGFR 19号外显子的缺失，可能是由于脑脊液检测的敏感性较低而产生了错误结果。如果作者能加上解决这些局限性的改善方案，就更好了。

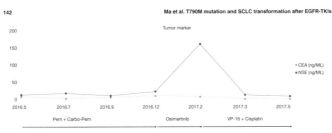

142　　　　　　　　　　　　　　　　Ma et al. T790M mutation and SCLC transformation after EGFR-TKIs

Figure 2 Predictive function of NSE for SCLC transformation. After osimertinib therapy was initiated, the levels of NSE in the serum gradually increased. After etoposide plus cisplatin chemotherapy, the levels of NSE sharply decreased. SCLC, small cell lung cancer; CEA, carcinoembryonic antigen; NSE, neuron-specific enolase; Pem, pemetrexed; Carbo, carboplatin; VP-16, etoposide.

alveolar type II cells may be common precursors of both lung adenocarcinoma and SCLC. Thus, EGFR-mutant lung cancers have the potential to transform into SCLCs during disease progression (16,17). Another hypothesis is that initial tumors consisted of mixed NSCLC and SCLC components. After treatment with EGFR-TKIs, the number of NSCLC decreased and the SCLC became dominant (16). This positive drug selection possibly depends on the tumor microenvironment in lesions in each organ, which results in spatial heterogeneity between lung and chest lesions.

条目11c

It has been reported that the rapid increase of tumor markers including NSE and pro-gastrin releasing-peptide (pro-GRP) during EGFR-TKI treatment are usually an indication of transformation from NSCLC to SCLC (18-20). In the present case, the remarkably increase in serum levels of NSE highlighted the necessity of repeat biopsy and suggested SCLC transformation (*Figure 2*).

条目11b

Recently, a retrospective study examined 58 NSCLC patients diagnosed with adenocarcinoma that transformed to SCLC after one or more EGFR-TKI treatments (21). Median time to transformation was 17.8 months (95% CI, 14.3 to 26.2 months). After transformation, both platinum-etoposide and taxanes yielded high response rates. Median OS after diagnosis was 31.5 months (95% CI, 24.8 to 41.3 months), whereas median survival after the time of SCLC transformation was 10.9 months (95% CI, 8.0 to 13.7 months). In our case, etoposide plus cisplatin chemotherapy yielded considerable response with a response of PR and a PFS of 4 months. The time from diagnosis to transformation was 24 months, and the OS of the patient was 29 months.

In summary, we experienced a case of concomitant mechanisms of drug-resistance via T790M mutation and transformation to SCLC. The dynamic changes among the specific mutations depend on drug-induced selection, which possibly led to drug-resistance. Overall, repeat biopsy is essential for patients whose disease progresses while they are receiving EGFR-TKIs so that appropriate treatment decisions can be made according to the diverse mechanisms of acquired resistance.

条目11d

Acknowledgments

Funding: None.

Footnote

Conflicts of Interest: The authors have no conflicts of interest to declare.

Ethical Statement: The authors are accountable for all aspects of the work in ensuring that questions related to the accuracy or integrity of any part of the work are appropriately investigated and resolved. Written informed consent was obtained from the patient for publication of this manuscript and any accompanying images.

Open Access Statement: This is an Open Access article distributed in accordance with the Creative Commons Attribution-NonCommercial-NoDerivs 4.0 International License (CC BY-NC-ND 4.0), which permits the non-commercial replication and distribution of the article with

　　Transl Lung Cancer Res 2020;9(1):139-143 | http://dx.doi.org/10.21037/tlcr.2020.01.07

条目11c：讨论　给出结论的科学依据，包括对可能原因的评估

详细总结了小细胞肺癌转化的3个可能机制。一是肺泡 II 型细胞是肺腺癌和小细胞肺癌的共同前体。因此，EGFR突变的肺癌有可能在疾病发展过程中转变为小细胞肺癌。二是最初的肿瘤由非小细胞肺癌和小细胞肺癌混合成分组成，用EGFR-TKIs治疗后，非小细胞肺癌的数量减少，小细胞肺癌成为主导。三是肿瘤标志物的快速增加通常是向小细胞肺癌转化的标志。但作者未能解释题目中的另一个结局，即获得性T790M突变的可能机制，这一点有待完善。

条目11b：讨论　引用参考文献以展开对相关医学文献的讨论

作者引用了一项包含58例腺癌患者的回顾性研究，该研究采用EGFR-TKI治疗后，患者均转变为小细胞肺癌，平均转化时间为17.8个月，平均生存期为31.5个月，而转化后的平均生存期为10.9个月。本病例的无进展生存期为4个月，从诊断到转变的时间为24个月，总生存期为29个月。如果作者能补充说明该患者生存期较长的可能原因会更好，因为这会是医生和患者最关心的问题，可以给未来遇到类似情况时如何提高生存期提供思路。

条目11d：讨论　用一个无参考文献的段落来给出结论，说明本病例报告的主要启示

报告到位。对于接受EGFR-TKIs治疗期间疾病进展的患者来说，重复活检是必不可少的，这样才能根据获得性耐药的不同机制作出适当的治疗决定。

条目12：患者观点　用1~2个段落分享患者对所接受的治疗的看法

如果可能，最好用1~2个段落分享患者对所接受的治疗的看法，但作者未提供。

条目13：知情同意　患者是否知情同意？如有需要，请提供知情同意书

根据期刊要求，作者需要尽可能在发表该病例前取得患者知情同意，但作者未说明。详见本书第二章相关内容。

Translational Lung Cancer Research, Vol 9, No 1 February 2020

143

the strict proviso that no changes or edits are made and the original work is properly cited (including links to both the formal publication through the relevant DOI and the license). See: https://creativecommons.org/licenses/by-nc-nd/4.0/.

References

1. Ohashi K, Maruvka YE, Michor F, et al. Epidermal growth factor receptor tyrosine kinase inhibitor-resistant disease. J Clin Oncol 2013;31:1070-80.
2. Chen D, Chu T, Chang Q, et al. The relationship between preliminary efficacy and prognosis after first-line EGFR tyrosine kinase inhibitor (EGFR-TKI) treatment of advanced non-small cell lung cancer. Ann Transl Med 2019;7:195.
3. Lettig L, Sahnane N, Pepe F, et al. EGFR T790M detection rate in lung adenocarcinomas at baseline using droplet digital PCR and validation by ultra-deep next generation sequencing. Transl Lung Cancer Res 2019;8:584-92.
4. Ma L, Chen R, Wang F, et al. EGFR L718Q mutation occurs without T790M mutation in a lung adenocarcinoma patient with acquired resistance to osimertinib. Ann Transl Med 2019;7:207.
5. Mok TS, Wu YL, Ahn MJ, et al. Osimertinib or Platinum-Pemetrexed in EGFR T790M-Positive Lung Cancer. N Engl J Med 2017;376:629-40.
6. Ricordel C, Friboulet L, Facchinetti F, et al. Molecular mechanisms of acquired resistance to third-generation EGFR-TKIs in EGFR T790M-mutant lung cancer. Ann Oncol 2018;29:i28-i37.
7. Lim SM, Syn NL, Cho BC, et al. Acquired resistance to EGFR targeted therapy in non-small cell lung cancer: Mechanisms and therapeutic strategies. Cancer Treat Rev 2018;65:1-10.
8. Riley DS, Barber MS, Kienle GS, et al. CARE 2013 Explanations and Elaborations: Reporting Guidelines for Case Reports. J Clin Epidemiol 2017;89:218-35.
9. Sequist LV, Waltman BA, Dias-Santagata D, et al. Genotypic and histological evolution of lung cancers acquiring resistance to EGFR inhibitors. Sci Transl Med 2011;3:75ra26.
10. Thress KS, Paweletz CP, Felip E, et al. Acquired EGFR C797S mutation mediates resistance to AZD9291 in non-small cell lung cancer harboring EGFR T790M. Nat Med 2015;21:560-2.
11. Kim TM, Song A, Kim DW, et al. Mechanisms of Acquired Resistance to AZD9291: A Mutation-Selective, Irreversible EGFR Inhibitor. J Thorac Oncol 2015;10:1736-44.
12. Ham JS, Kim S, Kim HK, et al. Two Cases of Small Cell Lung Cancer Transformation from EGFR Mutant Adenocarcinoma During AZD9291 Treatment. J Thorac Oncol 2016;11:e1-4.
13. Li L, Wang H, Li C, et al. Transformation to small-cell carcinoma as an acquired resistance mechanism to AZD9291: A case report. Oncotarget 2017;8:18609-14.
14. Iijima Y, Hirotsu Y, Mochizuki H, et al. Dynamic Changes and Drug-Induced Selection of Resistant Clones in a Patient With EGFR-Mutated Adenocarcinoma That Acquired T790M Mutation and Transformed to Small-Cell Lung Cancer. Clin Lung Cancer 2018;19:e843-7.
15. Ali G, Bruno R, Giordano M, et al. Small cell lung cancer transformation and the T790M mutation: A case report of two acquired mechanisms of TKI resistance detected in a tumor rebiopsy and plasma sample of EGFR-mutant lung adenocarcinoma. Oncol Lett 2016;12:4009-12.
16. Oser MG, Niederst MJ, Sequist LV, et al. Transformation from non-small-cell lung cancer to small-cell lung cancer: molecular drivers and cells of origin. Lancet Oncol 2015;16:e165-72.
17. Shi X, Duan H, Liu X, et al. Genetic alterations and protein expression in combined small cell lung cancers and small cell lung cancers arising from lung adenocarcinoma after therapy with tyrosine kinase inhibitors. Oncotarget 2016;7:34240-9.
18. Zhang Y, Li XY, Tang Y, et al. Rapid increase of serum neuron specific enolase level and tachyphylaxis of EGFR-tyrosine kinase inhibitor indicate small cell lung cancer transformation from EGFR positive lung adenocarcinoma? Lung Cancer 2013;81:302-5.
19. Liu Y. Small cell lung cancer transformation from EGFR-mutated lung adenocarcinoma: A case report and literatures review. Cancer Biol Ther 2018;19:445-9.
20. Norkowski E, Ghigna MR, Lacroix L, et al. Small-cell carcinoma in the setting of pulmonary adenocarcinoma: new insights in the era of molecular pathology. J Thorac Oncol 2013;8:1265-71.
21. Marcoux N, Gettinger SN, O'Kane G, et al. EGFR-Mutant Adenocarcinomas That Transform to Small-Cell Lung Cancer and Other Neuroendocrine Carcinomas: Clinical Outcomes. J Clin Oncol 2019;37:278-85.

Cite this article as: Ma S, He Z, Fu H, Wang L, Wu X, Zhang Z, Wang Q. Dynamic changes of acquired T790M mutation and small cell lung cancer transformation in a patient with EGFR-mutant adenocarcinoma after first- and third-generation EGFR-TKIs: a case report. Transl Lung Cancer Res 2020;9(1):139-143. doi: 10.21037/tlcr.2020.01.07

 Transl Lung Cancer Res 2020;9(1):139-143 | http://dx.doi.org/10.21037/tlcr.2020.01.07

第二篇病例报告案例解析

Case Report

条目1

Pancreatic INI1-deficient undifferentiated rhabdoid carcinoma achieves complete clinical response on gemcitabine and nab-paclitaxel following immediate progression on FOLFIRINOX: a case report

Daniel A. King[1], Smruti Rahalkar[1], David B. Bingham[2], George A. Fisher[1]

[1]Department of Medicine, Stanford University, Stanford, CA, USA; [2]Department of Pathology, Stanford University, Stanford, CA, USA
Correspondence to: Daniel A. King, George A. Fisher. Department of Medicine, Division of Oncology, Stanford University, 875 Blake Wilbur Drive, Stanford, CA 94305, USA. Email: danking@stanford.edu; georgeaf@stanford.edu.

条目3a

条目3b 3c

条目2

条目3d

Abstract: Introduction: INI1-deficient undifferentiated rhabdoid carcinoma is a rare pancreatic carcinoma for which the optimal treatment is unknown. Pancreatic ductal adenocarcinoma, the most common histology of pancreas cancer, is treated with combination chemotherapy in the advanced setting, a strategy supported by strong evidence in well powered studies. In patients with excellent performance status, first-line treatment usually consists of the three-drug regimen FOLFIRINOX, with the combination of gemcitabine with nab-paclitaxel, typically less toxic than the three-drug regimen, reserved for second-line therapy. Given the lack of published reports describing treatment outcomes for patients with rare forms of pancreatic cancer, the same treatment approach used for pancreatic ductal adenocarcinoma is typically employed. Observation: This case describes a patient with metastatic pancreatic INI1-deficient undifferentiated rhabdoid carcinoma who was primarily resistant to FOLFIRINOX therapy but who then achieved an immediate, marked and sustained response to gemcitabine with nab-paclitaxel. Conclusion: Given the lack of data informing on optimal management of INI1-deficient pancreatic undifferentiated carcinoma, and the exceptional response achieved by gemcitabine with nab-paclitaxel, this case report highlights a surprising and potentially informative anecdote. Additional studies are needed to confirm responses observed in this report which when taken together may strongly influence first-line therapy choice for this rare malignancy. Given the difficult in acquiring sufficient numbers of these rare histologies in any one institution, multi-institution collaboration in studying outcomes of rare pancreatic malignancies is likely essential.

Keywords: INI1-deficient undifferentiated rhabdoid carcinoma; sarcomatoid undifferentiated carcinoma; pancreatic cancer; case report

Submitted Oct 31, 2020. Accepted for publication Jan 17, 2021.
doi: 10.21037/jgo-20-478
View this article at: http://dx.doi.org/10.21037/jgo-20-478

条目4

Introduction

The optimal treatment of the rare malignancy INI1-deficient undifferentiated rhabdoid carcinoma is not known. This report describes a case of INI1-deficient undifferentiated rhabdoid carcinoma that achieved an exceptional response to gemcitabine with paclitaxel despite immediate progression on FOLFIRINOX.

We present the following article in accordance with the CARE reporting checklist (available at: http://dx.doi.org/10.21037/jgo-20-478).

Case presentation

条目5a 5b

A 59-year-old woman presented to the emergency room in March 2019 with acute abdominal pain (*Figure 1*). She was in otherwise good health, and past medical history

J Gastrointest Oncol 2021;12(2):874-879 | http://dx.doi.org/10.21037/jgo-20-478

条目1：标题　写明最初的诊断或干预关注点，其后加上"case report"

作者用PICOS方式拟定标题，并突出了最主要的点：P——胰腺INI1缺陷未分化横纹肌瘤，I——一线三药联合用药方案FOLFIRINOX后，二线使用吉西他滨联合纳布–紫杉醇，O——一线治疗方案后的快速进展与二线治疗方案后的完全临床反应，S——病例报告。

条目2：关键词　2~5个点明该病例报告的诊断或干预的关键词，包括"case report"

作者病例报告的关键词未遗漏case report，但另外3个关键词全是PICOS中P

的信息。笔者认为这则病例报告最值得关注的点是吉西他滨的特殊反应，所以可以在关键词中加入I的信息，使此文能更多维度地被检索到。

条目3a：摘要　这个案例有什么独特之处，它对科学文献有什么贡献？

报告到位。作者不只是指出INI1缺陷的未分化横纹肌瘤比较罕见，还重点强调了当前仍然缺乏最佳治疗方案，而该患者在二线治疗后取得了完全的临床反应，这是亮点和特点。

条目3b：摘要　重要临床发现
条目3c：摘要　主要诊断、治疗干预和结局

作者报道了患者的诊断、治疗方案、临床结局，以及最主要的临床发现，但未涵盖患者的一般信息，包括年龄、性别等，需要补充完整。

条目3d：摘要　结论　　该病例的主要收获是什么？

报告到位。作者主要强调了在当前缺乏最佳治疗方案的情况下，吉西他滨联合纳布–紫杉醇的特殊反应，以及这个发现的临床意义——可能会影响这种罕见疾病的一线治疗选择。另外，作者对下一步工作也提出了建议——倡导多中心合作来获得足够数量的病例以进一步评估此病例的发现。

条目4：引言　用1~2个段落总结为何该病例是独一无二的

作者介绍了INI1缺陷的未分化横纹肌瘤的罕见性和缺乏最佳治疗方法，篇幅短，一篇参考文献都没有用到，介绍苍白无力，可以说徒有"引言"之名。虽然作者再次强调此病例取得了完全临床反应，解决了临床问题，来吸引读者读下去，但作者没有发挥"引言"的介绍和铺垫作用，即没有阐述疾病的严重性、当前具体有哪些治疗方案、这些治疗方案的疗效、二线治疗方案后有没有类似取得完全临床反应的案例。

条目5a：患者信息　去除患者身份的具体信息
条目5b：患者信息　主诉和症状

报告到位。报告了年龄、性别这些与疾病相关的信息，以及患者主诉（急性腹痛）。

条目7

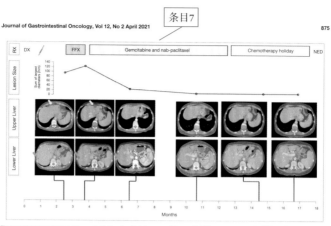

Journal of Gastrointestinal Oncology, Vol 12, No 2 April 2021

875

Figure 1 Treatment timeline. The x-axis displays the clinical course, with rows signifying: treatments received (Rx), radiographic burden of disease measured by calculating the sum of the maximal tumor dimensions of each liver lesion (Lesions Size), and characteristic lesions displayed (Upper Liver; Lower Liver; yellow and blue arrows). Initiation of gemcitabine and nab-paclitaxel led to an immediate and sustained decrease in tumor burden.

条目5c、5d

consisted only of a chondrosarcoma of the cranium, diagnosed in 2013, which was resected, radiated, and remained in remission through surveillance. There was no significant family medical history. On presentation in 2019, CT demonstrated a mass with solid and cystic components in the tail of the pancreas with no evidence of metastatic disease. FDG-PET showed intense uptake (SUV 12) in the pancreatic mass and no evidence of metastases. An EUS-guided FNA biopsy was highly suspicious for carcinoma. Both CEA and CA19-9 were within normal limits.

条目6

In April 2019, she underwent a robotic distal pancreatectomy with findings of a 1.6 cm invasive carcinoma with negative margins but with lymphovascular and perineural invasion and 1 of 35 nodes with malignant involvement. Surgical pathology review demonstrated sheets of monomorphic epithelioid cells with eosinophilic cytoplasm and a faint rhabdoid appearance but without glandular architecture, thus prompting consideration of a wide differential of non-adenocarcinoma neoplasms. Synaptophysin and chromogranin were negative, providing no support for neuroendocrine differentiation.

There was no expression of p63, lending no support for myoepithelial or squamous differentiation. ERG and CD34 were negative, providing no support for vascular differentiation. HMB45 negativity ruled out perivascular epithelioid cell tumor (PEComa). Lack of Sox-10/S100 and CD45RB expression, refuted metastatic melanoma or hematolymphoid differentiation, respectively. Given the patient's prior chondrosarcoma, that histology was compared to the pancreatic specimen, but the morphology was not similar. CK19 and CK7 were positive while CDX2 was negative, consistent with a pancreatic neoplasm. Immunohistochemical staining was broadly positive for pan-cytokeratin CKmix, consistent with epithelial differentiation. Stains for INI1 (SMARCB1) demonstrated a complete loss of nuclear expression in the neoplastic cells (*Figure 2*). Additional molecular studies showed intact mismatch repair proteins, PD-L1 expression with CPS of 20, and HER2 IHC was negative. Targeted tumor mutational profiling with the Stanford Tumor Actionable Mutation Panel identified a *KRAS* G12D mutation and variants of unknown significance in *EPHA2* C376F and

 J Gastrointest Oncol 2021;12(2):874-879 | http://dx.doi.org/10.21037/jgo-20-478

条目8a、8b、8c、8d

条目5c：患者信息 医疗、家庭和社会心理史，包括相关的遗传信息
条目5d：患者信息 过去的相关干预措施及结果

报告到位。报告了患者的既往史——2013年诊断为颅骨软骨肉瘤，并行手术切除和放疗，且治疗后病情稳定，患者无相关家族史。

条目6：临床发现 描述重要的检查和重要的临床发现

报告到位。2019年CT显示胰腺尾部有一肿块，无转移症状。FDG-PET显示肿块有异常高的摄取率，活检高度怀疑是癌细胞。

条目7：时间轴 以时间轴的形式组织诊治照护信息，包括历史信息和当前信息

这是本书第二章中关于时间轴的"良好报告示范"，详见第21页解析。另外，作者也在文章中有对应年月的相关陈述，这很好。

条目 8a、8b、8c、8d

a *KDR* L1095 frameshift, consistent with a low tumor mutational burden. Multigene testing for inherited mutations identified no abnormalities. The overall findings were that of a stage IIb (pT1c N1 M0) primary pancreatic INI1-deficient undifferentiated rhabdoid carcinoma.

Prior to a planned course of adjuvant chemotherapy, a CT in June 2019 demonstrated multiple [6–7] new liver metastases, the largest of which was 1.9 cm. FNA of one of the lesions confirmed metastatic disease of similar histology. An attempt to grow organoids from the biopsy

 J Gastrointest Oncol 2021;12(2):874-879 | http://dx.doi.org/10.21037/jgo-20-478

条目8a：诊断评估 诊断检查，如体格检查、实验室检查、影像学检查、调查
条目8b：诊断评估 诊断方面的挑战，如是否有条件开展检查、费用或文化挑战
条目8c：诊断评估 诊断，包括鉴别诊断
条目8d：诊断评估 预后，如肿瘤学中的分期（如适用）

报告到位。这是一则诊断有挑战的案例，所以作者详细交代了诊断和鉴别诊断的经过，并提供了重要的诊断测试结果和疾病分期。

患者接受胰腺切除术，发现1.6 cm的浸润性癌，边缘阴性，但有淋巴管和神经周围浸润，35个淋巴结中有1个呈恶性。病理检查结果显示，单形上皮细胞有嗜酸细胞质和微弱的横纹肌外观，但没有腺体结构。突触素和嗜铬粒蛋白阴性，不支持神经内分泌的分化。没有p63的表达，不支持肌上皮细胞或鳞状细胞的分化。ERG和CD34为阴性，不支持血管分化。HMB45阴性，排除了血管周围上皮细胞瘤。缺乏Sox-10/S100和CD45RB的表达，分别否定了转移性黑色素瘤或血淋巴分化。鉴于患者之前患有软骨肉瘤，将该组织学标本与胰腺标本进行了比较，但形态并不相似。CK19和CK7为阳性，而CDX2为阴性，与胰腺肿瘤一致。免疫组织化学染色显示泛细胞角蛋白CKmix呈广泛阳性，与上皮细胞分化一致。INI1的染色显示肿瘤细胞的核表达完全消失。其他分子研究显示错配修复蛋白完好，PD–L1表达，CPS为20，而HER2 IHC为阴性。同时，在EPHA2 C376F中存在KRAS G12D突变和意义未知的变异，以及KDR L1095移码突变，与低肿瘤突变负荷一致。遗传性突变的多基因检测未发现异常。最终，诊断为Ⅱb期的原发性胰腺INI1缺陷的未分化横纹肌瘤。2019年6月，疾病进展，CT显示有多个新的肝转移灶，其中最大的直径有1.9 cm。

Journal of Gastrointestinal Oncology, Vol 12, No 2 April 2021

条目 9a、8d

was unsuccessful.

She then received three doses of mFOLFIRINOX but due to progressive increase in right upper quadrant pain, a CT scan was ordered prior to a planned 4th dose, which demonstrated an increase in size and number of liver metastases (*Figure 1*) warranting change in therapy.

条目 9c、8d

In July of 2019, she was switched to gemcitabine 850 mg/m² with nab-paclitaxel 100 mg/m². Treatment on cycle 1 day 15 was held due to cytopenia. A short interval scan in August 2019, after receiving day 1 and day 8 of treatment, showed no new hepatic lesions and size stability of all known liver lesions. Treatment frequency was reduced to every other week dosing on account of the cytopenia.

条目 8d、12

Following two months of therapy, she had a dramatic clinical improvement, reporting that her abdominal pain had decreased to a level of 1–2 out of 10 and she had stopped taking all analgesics. She said that she felt as well as she did before her illness. Follow-up CT CAP in October 2019 showed marked reduction in the size of multiple hepatic metastases. She continued biweekly therapy. By November 2019, her abdominal pain had resolved completely. She developed peripheral neuropathy for which the nab-paclitaxel dose was reduced, and a rash, which was managed with prednisone. CT scan in December 2019 showed continued response, with all remaining liver disease subcentimeter in size. She started planning

条目 10d

条目 8d、10b

a long-distance vacation. By late January, CT no longer identified any lesions in the liver. In March of 2020, she began a chemotherapy holiday, and at scan and follow-up in August 2020, she remained without radiographic or clinical evidence of disease, and continues on surveillance off treatment at the time of submission.

All procedures performed in studies involving human participants were in accordance with the ethical standards of the institutional and/or national research committee(s) and with the Helsinki Declaration (as revised in 2013). Written informed consent was obtained from the patient.

条目 13

Discussion

The histologic classification of undifferentiated carcinoma is complex. Undifferentiated rhabdoid carcinoma of the pancreas is quite rare with fewer than 100 cases reported in the literature (1). According to the latest WHO classification system, these tumors fall within the broader category of sarcomatoid undifferentiated carcinoma (2). Agaimy *et al.* have further subtyped undifferentiated rhabdoid carcinomas into two groups, a pleomorphic

variant which tends to have KRAS alterations, and a monomorphic variant (such as the tumor discussed in this report) which tends to be INI1-deficient (1). Few data inform optimal treatment strategies for these very rare malignancies. A case report demonstrating complete response to a paclitaxel-containing regimen in pleomorphic variant undifferentiated pancreatic carcinoma was published in 2010 (3). SMARCB1/INI1-deficiency is a recently recognized molecular hallmark of renal medullary carcinoma (4), where paclitaxel-containing combinations have shown partial (5) and complete responses (6). To our knowledge, the work presented here is the first publication describing the clinical course and response to chemotherapy in a patient with metastatic INI1-deficient undifferentiated rhabdoid carcinoma.

Chromatin accessibility is a tightly regulated process and an integral determinant of gene expression. Disruption of chromatin remodeling can promote tumorigenesis (7,8). The gene *INI1*, also known as *SMARB1*, for SWI/SNF-related matrix-associated actin-dependent regulator of chromatin subfamily B member 1, encodes for proteins involved in relieving repressive chromatin structures, thus acting as a tumor suppressor gene (9). Its carcinogenicity is in part linked to is dysregulation of cyclin-dependent kinase inhibitor p16, Wnt signaling, and E2F factors, among others (10). Following diagnosis in any age or organ, nearly all SMARCB1/INI1-deficient malignancies typically follow an aggressive clinical pattern and have a poor prognosis (1).

On presentation, the patient was 59 years old, with excellent performance status after her operation. Lacking specific guidelines to inform therapy selection in this rare histology, chemotherapy was chosen based on extrapolation for pancreatic ductal adenocarcinoma. Thus, first-line therapy with FOLFIRINOX was chosen, which is associated with a median overall survival of 11 months in patients with metastatic pancreatic adenocarcinoma (11). The cancer immediately progressed through first line therapy. Gemcitabine with nab-paclitaxel was chosen for second-line therapy, and the patient had an immediate response. The lack of long-term follow-up is a limitation of this case report. Nevertheless, the response thus far achieved was remarkable: two studies have explored the response rate of second-line gemcitabine with nab-paclitaxel in metastatic pancreatic ductal adenocarcinoma following FOLFIRINOX therapy: (I) in a study of 30 patients, including 11/30 (37%) who had progressive disease on FOLFIRINOX, there were 0/30 patients on gemcitabine with nab-paclitaxel who then achieved a complete response

条目 11a

J Gastrointest Oncol 2021;12(2):874-879 | http://dx.doi.org/10.21037/jgo-20-478

条目9a：治疗干预　治疗干预的类型，如药物、手术、预防、自我护理等

条目8d：诊断评估　预后，如肿瘤学中的分期（如适用）

　　作者报告了患者接受的3个剂量的mFOLFIRINOX化疗，但没有描述具体药物名称、剂量和用法。作者对疾病预后报告到位：由于右上腹疼痛逐渐加重，在第4个剂量之前，再次CT扫描显示肝转移灶的大小和数量增加，疾病进一步进展。

条目9c：治疗干预　治疗干预的变化，需要提供改变理由

条目8d：诊断评估　预后，如肿瘤学中的分期（如适用）

　　报告到位。报告了更换治疗方案的原因——疾病进展，以及具体后续治疗方案——2019年7月，改用吉西他滨和纳布-紫杉醇（有明确的剂量）。2019年8月，在接受第1天和第8天的治疗后，扫描显示没有出现新的肝脏病变，病变稳定。但是由于细胞减少，第1个化疗周期第15天治疗被搁置，于是再次更改治疗方案，用药频率降至每2周1次。

条目8d：诊断评估　预后，如肿瘤学中的分期（如适用）
条目12：患者观点　应用1~2个段落分享患者对所接受治疗的看法

　　报告到位：2个月的治疗后，患者临床症状有明显的改善，主诉腹痛减轻，且停止服用镇痛药，感觉良好。这里描述了患者的感受，可以从患者的视角更多维度地展现病例。2019年10月，CT显示肝转移灶明显缩小，继续维持化疗。2019年11月，腹痛完全缓解。

条目10d：随访和结局　不良和预期之外的事件

　　报告到位。患者出现周围神经病变和皮疹，用泼尼松处理。作者客观描述了不良反应和具体处理措施。

条目8d：诊断评估　预后，如肿瘤学中的分期（如适用）
条目10b：随访和结局　重要的后续诊断和其他测试结果

　　报告到位。2019年12月，CT显示持续缓解，肝转移灶逐渐缩小。2020年1月，CT未发现肝脏任何病变。2020年3月，停止化疗。截至撰稿，作者对患者的随访检查未发现疾病的放射学或临床证据。该病例报告有始有终，详略得当，全面描述了不同时间点上患者的疾病进展、相应的治疗改变，以及随访结局，值得借鉴。

条目13：知情同意　患者是否知情同意？如有需要，请提供知情同意书

　　报告到位。作者表示，已获得患者的书面知情同意。

条目11a：讨论　对本病例报告的优点和局限性进行科学讨论

　　缺乏长期随访是本病例报告的一个局限，虽然对患者进行了随访，但作者没有回避时间较短这个问题。此项是写作时较易忽略的问题，可参见本书第二章的详细说明。

条目11b

and only 4/30 (13%) achieved a partial response (12); and (II) among 57 patients, including 16 of 57 (28%) who had progressive disease on FOLFIRINOX, there were 0 of 57 patients achieving a complete response and only 22 of 57 (39%) achieving a partial response (13). Thus, while primary refractoriness to FOLFIRINOX is not rare (37%, and 27%), achieving a complete response to gemcitabine with nab-paclitaxel has not been previously reported and thus this case is exceptional.

条目11c

The underlying mechanism explaining the complete clinical response to gemcitabine with nab-paclitaxel despite rapid progression on FOLFIRINOX is not clear. We speculate that the excellent response achieved with gemcitabine and nab-paclitaxel may be related to the different mechanism of action of the latter, which may better synergize with INI1 deficiency-mediated defects in chromatin remodeling. We note an established link between defects in chromatin remodeling and mitotic spindle function (14), suggesting a role for synergism or synthetic lethality when combining INI1 deficient neoplasms with microtubule inhibitors. Combining HDAC inhibitors with other therapeutics in pancreatic cancer is an area of active investigation (15), but has met with limited success. For example, trials in pancreatic ductal adenocarcinoma using HDAC inhibitors along with gemcitabine have largely been disappointing (8). It has been shown that HDAC inhibitors potentiate topoisomerase I-mediated DNA damage (16) and exploiting the rationale that HDAC inhibitors may sensitize tumors to topoisomerase inhibitors is an area of active study (17). As an alternative explanation, we note that while CPS score is not commonly used as a predictive biomarker in pancreatic cancer, the CPS score in this case was 20, suggesting a robust degree of immunogenicity of the tumor; perhaps this PD-L1 staining immune compartment primed an immune response for second-line therapy. Ultimately, a greater mechanistic understanding is needed to identify predictive biomarkers of response for this rare pancreatic neoplasm.

条目11d

In conclusion, while the optimal treatment for INI1-deficient undifferentiated rhabdoid carcinoma of the pancreas is not known, this clinical case report highlights an exceptional response to gemcitabine with nab-paclitaxel, despite initial failure of FOLFIRINOX, which may rightfully influence first-line treatment selection in this rare malignancy.

Acknowledgments

Funding: None.

Footnote

Reporting Checklist: The authors have completed the CARE reporting checklist. Available at: http://dx.doi.org/10.21037/jgo-20-478

Conflicts of Interest: All authors have completed the ICMJE uniform disclosure form (available at: http://dx.doi.org/10.21037/jgo-20-478). George Fisher reports personal fees from Merck, Taiho, Roche, Terumo and Ipsen; and has served data safety monitoring boards for Astra Zeneca, Hutchison Pharma and Cytom X and Silenseed. The other authors have no conflict of interests to disclose.

Ethical Statement: The authors are accountable for all aspects of the work in ensuring that questions related to the accuracy or integrity of any part of the work are appropriately investigated and resolved. All procedures performed in studies involving human participants were in accordance with the ethical standards of the institutional and/or national research committee(s) and with the Helsinki Declaration (as revised in 2013). Written informed consent was obtained from the patient.

References

1. Agaimy A, Haller F, Frohnauer J, et al. Pancreatic undifferentiated rhabdoid carcinoma: KRAS alterations and SMARCB1 expression status define two subtypes. Mod Pathol 2015;28:248-60.
2. Nagtegaal ID, Odze RD, Klimstra D, et al. The 2019 WHO classification of tumours of the digestive system. Histopathology 2020;76:182-8.
3. Wakatsuki T, Irisawa A, Imamura H, et al. Complete response of anaplastic pancreatic carcinoma to paclitaxel treatment selected by chemosensitivity testing. Int J Clin Oncol 2010;15:310-3.
4. Jia L, Carlo MI, Khan H, et al. Distinctive mechanisms underlie the loss of SMARCB1 protein expression in renal

J Gastrointest Oncol 2021;12(2):874-879 | http://dx.doi.org/10.21037/jgo-20-478

条目11b：讨论　引用参考文献以展开对相关医学文献的讨论

报告到位。作者没有回避和该病例类似的案例，而是将两个极为类似的案例与该病例进行了比较。作者指出，另外两个案例中，吉西他滨联合纳布-紫杉醇对转移性胰腺导管腺癌在经FOLFIRINOX方案治疗后的反应率，均未发现任何患者获得完全反应，而该病例患者出现了完全反应。

条目11c：讨论　给出结论的科学依据，包括对可能原因的评估

报告到位。作者对该患者二线治疗后获得完全反应提出了两个详细的假说

且有科学依据——参考文献14~17。假说一，吉西他滨联合纳布-紫杉醇取得的良好反应可能与纳布-紫杉醇的作用机制不同有关，它能更好地协同INI1缺陷介导的染色质重塑缺陷。假说二，该病例的CPS评分为20，表明肿瘤的免疫原性程度很强，也许这种PD-L1染色的免疫区块启动了二线治疗的免疫反应。

条目11d：讨论　用一个无参考文献的段落来给出结论，说明本病例报告的主要启示

报告到位。作者总结了本病例的经验，并指出该发现可能会影响INI1缺乏的未分化胰腺横纹肌瘤的一线治疗选择。作者措辞严谨，没有夸大该病例的临床意义。

Journal of Gastrointestinal Oncology, Vol 12, No 2 April 2021　　　　879

medullary carcinoma: morphologic and molecular analysis of 20 cases. Mod Pathol 2019;32:1329-43.

5. Gangireddy V gopala reddy, Liles GB, Sostre GD, et al. Response of metastatic renal medullary carcinoma to carboplatinum and paclitaxel chemotherapy. Clin Genitourin Cancer 2012;10:134-9.

6. Walsh A, Kelly DR, Vaid YN, et al. Complete response to carboplatin, gemcitabine, and paclitaxel in a patient with advanced metastatic renal medullary carcinoma. Pediatr Blood Cancer 2010;55:1217-20.

7. Wolffe AP. Chromatin remodeling: Why it is important in cancer. Oncogene 2001;20:2988-90.

8. Hessmann E, Johnsen SA, Siveke JT, et al. Epigenetic treatment of pancreatic cancer: Is there a therapeutic perspective on the horizon? Gut 2017;66:168-79.

9. Hollmann TJ, Hornick JL. INI1-deficient tumors: Diagnostic features and molecular genetics. Am J Surg Pathol 2011;35:e47-63.

10. Kalimuthu SN, Chetty R. Gene of the month: SMARCB1. J Clin Pathol 2016;69:484-9.

11. Conroy T, Desseigne F, Ychou M, et al. FOLFIRINOX

12. Mita N, Iwashita T, Uemura S, et al. Second-Line Gemcitabine Plus Nab-Paclitaxel for Patients with Unresectable Advanced Pancreatic Cancer after First-Line FOLFIRINOX Failure. J Clin Med 2019;8:761.

13. Portal A, Pernot S, Tougeron D, et al. Nab-paclitaxel plus gemcitabine for metastatic pancreatic adenocarcinoma after Folfirinox failure: An AGEO prospective multicentre cohort. Br J Cancer 2015;113:989-95.

14. Giaccia AJ. A New Chromatin-Cytoskeleton Link in Cancer. Mol Cancer Res 2016;14:1173-5.

15. Baretti M, Ahuja N, Azad NS. Targeting the epigenome of pancreatic cancer for therapy: challenges and opportunities. Ann Pancreat Cancer 2019;2:18.

16. Thurn KT, Thomas S, Moore A, et al. Rational therapeutic combinations with histone deacetylase inhibitors for the treatment of cancer. Future Oncol 2011;7:263-83.

17. Seo YH. Dual Inhibitors Against Topoisomerases and Histone Deacetylases. J Cancer Prev 2015;20:85-91.

Cite this article as: King DA, Rahalkar S, Bingham DB, Fisher GA. Pancreatic INI1-deficient undifferentiated rhabdoid carcinoma achieves complete clinical response on gemcitabine and nab-paclitaxel following immediate progression on FOLFIRINOX: a case report. J Gastrointest Oncol 2021;12(2):874-879. doi: 10.21037/jgo-20-478

第三篇病例系列案例解析

Case Report

条目1

Safety of lorlatinib following alectinib-induced pneumonitis in two patients with *ALK*-rearranged non-small cell lung cancer: a case series

Nathaniel J. Myall[1], Amy Q. Lei[2], Heather A. Wakelee[1]

[1]Division of Oncology, Stanford Cancer Institute, Stanford, CA, USA; [2]Division of Oncology, Kaiser Permanente Santa Clara Medical Center, Santa Clara, CA, USA

Correspondence to: Dr. Heather A. Wakelee, MD. Stanford Cancer Institute, 875 Blake Wilbur Drive, Stanford, CA 94305, USA. Email: hwakelee@stanford.edu.

条目3a

Abstract: Drug-induced interstitial lung disease (DI-ILD) is a rare adverse event associated with targeted therapies that inhibit the anaplastic lymphoma kinase (ALK) protein. Although newer-generation ALK inhibitors such as alectinib significantly improve survival in metastatic *ALK*-rearranged non-small cell lung cancer (NSCLC), the risk of DI-ILD is similar to that of earlier-generation therapies. Lorlatinib is a third-generation ALK inhibitor that is active in patients with metastatic NSCLC whose tumors have developed secondary resistance to alectinib. While it is associated with low rates of DI-ILD in initial phase 1/2 clinical trials, the safety of lorlatinib in patients with a history of DI-ILD has not been well-described. In this case series, we therefore report two patients with metastatic *ALK*-rearranged NSCLC who each tolerated

条目3b 3c

lorlatinib following recovery from alectinib-related DI-ILD. Both cases were notable for the acute onset of dyspnea, hypoxia, and diffuse ground-glass opacities within one month of initiating alectinib. With no alternative etiology of pneumonitis identified, both patients were treated empirically for grade 3 DI-ILD with corticosteroids and discontinuation of alectinib. Following rapid clinical recovery and eventual radiographic resolution of opacities, each patient was started on lorlatinib at the time of cancer progression, with neither person developing symptoms or radiographic findings consistent with recurrent DI-ILD. In the following series, we describe these two cases in greater detail and discuss their significance within the context

条目2

of the prior literature. While further descriptions are needed, our experience suggests that lorlatinib may be a safe therapeutic option in some patients who have recovered from DI-ILD.

Keywords: Non-small cell lung cancer (NSCLC); anaplastic lymphoma kinase (ALK); interstitial lung disease; alectinib; lorlatinib; case series

条目3d

Submitted Apr 19, 2020. Accepted for publication Aug 28, 2020.
doi: 10.21037/tlcr-20-564
View this article at: http://dx.doi.org/10.21037/tlcr-20-564

Introduction

条目4

Alectinib is a second-generation tyrosine kinase inhibitor (TKI) that significantly improves progression-free survival compared to crizotinib in untreated patients with metastatic, *anaplastic lymphoma kinase (ALK)*-rearranged non-small cell lung cancer (NSCLC) (1). Like other ALK inhibitors, it is associated in rare cases with serious adverse events such as drug-induced interstitial lung disease (DI-ILD) or pneumonitis. Because DI-ILD is thought to represent a

potential side-effect of all ALK inhibitors, switching from alectinib to another targeted therapy within the same class requires careful consideration in those patients who have a history of DI-ILD.

Lorlatinib is a novel, third-generation ALK inhibitor that has activity against acquired *ALK* resistance mutations (e.g., G1202R) and has been associated with low rates (<1%) of DI-ILD in phase 1/2 clinical trials (2-4). These previous studies, however, specifically excluded patients who had a

Transl Lung Cancer Res 2021;10(1):487-495 | http://dx.doi.org/10.21037/tlcr-20-564

条目1：标题　写明最初的诊断或干预关注点，其后加上"case report"

报告到位。作者用PICOS方式拟定标题，并突出了最主要的点，即P——ALK重组的非小细胞肺癌患者，I——艾乐替尼及劳拉替尼，O——艾乐替尼诱导的间质性肺炎及换用劳拉替尼后间质性肺炎未再复发，S——病例系列（当文章是病例系列而非单个病例报告时要知道灵活变通）。

条目2：关键词 **2~5个点明该病例报告的诊断或干预的关键词，包括"case report"**

报告到位。关键词体现出了标题中部分PICOS，且作者未遗漏 case series（当文章为病例系列而非单个病例报告时，关键词最好用case series）。

条目3a：摘要 **这个案例有什么独特之处，它对科学文献有什么贡献？**

报告到位。作者指出对于劳拉替尼在药物诱导的间质性肺病（drug-induced interstitial lung disease，DI-ILD）患者中的安全性还没有很好的研究，而这个病例则可以填补这一研究空缺。

条目3b：摘要 **主要症状和（或）重要的临床发现**
条目3c：摘要 **主要诊断、治疗干预和结局**

作者介绍了患者的临床发现、主要干预和结局。他们对使用艾乐替尼后出现DI-ILD的患者采用皮质类固醇治疗，并停用艾乐替尼。好转后，患者开始接受劳拉替尼治疗，之后两位患者都没有出现DI-ILD复发。如果作者能再介绍患者其他的重要信息会更好，比如年龄、肺癌的分期等。

条目3d：摘要 **结论——该病例的主要收获是什么？**

报告到位。对于一些DI-ILD恢复的患者，劳拉替尼可能是一种安全的治疗选择。

条目4：引言 **用1~2个段落总结为何该病例是独一无二的**

作者首先介绍了艾乐替尼会引起DI-ILD，对于有DI-ILD病史的患者来说，药物的转换需要仔细考虑。接着，作者提到劳拉替尼对获得性ALK耐药突变具有活性，且发现与DI-ILD呈弱相关，同时强调了3~4级DI-ILD患者的治疗方法和劳拉替尼在DI-ILD方面的安全性仍不清楚。所以有必要进行研究，引出该病例可以填补此"安全性仍不清楚"的空缺，突出其独特性和价值。

条目6、8a

history of grade 3–4 interstitial lung disease, and thus, both the optimal treatment of such patients and the full safety profile of lorlatinib with respect DI-ILD remain unclear. To begin addressing some of these unanswered questions, we describe two patients with *ALK*-rearranged NSCLC who each safely tolerated lorlatinib without recrudescent symptoms following recovery from grade 3 DI-ILD secondary to alectinib. We present the article in accordance with the CARE reporting checklist (available at http://dx.doi.org/10.21037/tlcr-20-564) (5).

Case presentation

Case #1

An 80-year-old Asian, non-smoking man with a history of stroke presented in 2018 with chest pain, fatigue, and weight

loss. A CT scan revealed a cavitary mass in the left lower lung measuring 6.5 cm × 4.3 cm × 3.3 cm without diffuse parenchymal disease (*Figure 1A*). PET-CT demonstrated additional hypermetabolic activity in the left hilar (SUV 6.8) and para-esophageal lymph nodes (SUV 4.4), bilateral adrenal glands (SUV 6.9), and right kidney (SUV 13.6). MRI of the brain revealed a punctate enhancing lesion in the right cerebellum, concerning for metastasis. Biopsy of the cavitary lung mass was consistent with a CK7+, TTF1+, CK20- lung adenocarcinoma with high PD-L1 expression (70%). Fluorescence in-situ hybridization (FISH) further revealed the presence of an *ALK* rearrangement.

Several weeks following the diagnosis of stage IV (cT3N2M1c) *ALK*-rearranged NSCLC, the patient was started on first-line alectinib 600 mg twice daily. On day 18 of therapy, he was admitted to the hospital with dyspnea and chest pain secondary to both multifocal pulmonary

条目8c、9a

条目5b

Transl Lung Cancer Res 2021;10(1):487-495 | http://dx.doi.org/10.21037/tlcr-20-564

条目5a、5c

第一个病例

条目5a：患者信息　去除患者身份的具体信息
条目5c：患者信息　医疗、家庭和社会心理史，包括相关的遗传信息

　　报告到位。报告了患者种族、年龄、性别、吸烟史与疾病相关的信息；患者有脑卒中既往史，2018年出现胸痛、疲劳和体重减轻。

条目6：临床发现　描述重要的检查和重要的临床发现
条目8a：诊断评估　诊断检查，如体格检查、实验室检查、影像学检查、调查

　　报告到位。详细描述了各种检查结果及临床发现，包括：CT扫描显示左下肺有一个空腔性肿块（大小）；PET–CT显示左肺和食道旁淋巴结、双侧肾上腺和右肾有高代谢活动；脑部MRI显示右侧小脑转移，肺部肿块的活检结果与肺腺癌一致；荧光原位杂交显示存在ALK重排。

条目8c：诊断评估　诊断，包括鉴别诊断
条目9a：治疗干预　治疗干预的类型，如药物、手术、预防、自我护理等

　　报告到位。患者最终被诊断为Ⅳ期ALK重组的非小细胞肺癌，开始接受一线艾乐替尼治疗，作者报告了该治疗的具体剂量和用法。

条目7

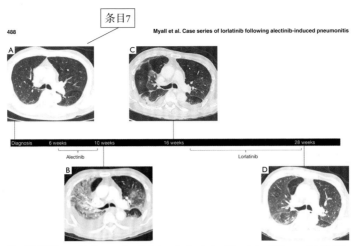

488 Myall et al. Case series of lorlatinib following alectinib-induced pneumonitis

Figure 1 Serial CT images of the chest were collected in the first patient from the time of diagnosis through follow-up on lorlatinib. At the time of presentation with NSCLC, no parenchymal abnormalities were observed aside from the primary tumor (not shown) (A). However, bilateral, diffuse ground-glass opacities and septal thickening became apparent 29 days after the initiation of alectinib when the patient developed worsening respiratory symptoms and hypoxia (B). Approximately 5 weeks after initiating corticosteroids and discontinuing alectinib for grade 4 DI-ILD, the previously seen parenchymal abnormalities were significantly improved (C). After 10 weeks on lorlatinib therapy, despite progression of NSCLC (not shown), only faint ground-glass opacities were visible compared to prior (D). NSCLC, non-small cell lung cancer; DI-ILD, drug-induced interstitial lung disease.

条目5b：患者信息　主诉和症状

患者在化疗的第18天，因呼吸困难和胸痛入院，继发于多灶性肺栓塞和大量左胸腔积液。

条目7：时间轴　以时间轴的形式组织诊治照护信息，包括历史信息和当前信息

作者报告了患者从确诊到随访整个期间的情况，包括患者使用艾乐替尼和劳拉替尼前后的影像学表现。由于除了停用艾乐替尼外，作者还采用了甲强龙来治疗DI-ILD，因此最好把甲强龙也加入时间轴中，否则容易将DI-ILD没有复发单纯地归功于停用艾乐替尼和换用劳拉替尼。另外，建议作者补上患者的随访结果。

条目9a：治疗干预　治疗干预的类型，如药物、手术、预防、自我护理等
条目8d：诊断评估　预后，如肿瘤学中的分期（如适用）

报告到位。进行抗凝治疗，放置留置胸腔导管，并继续使用艾乐替尼。

Translational Lung Cancer Research, Vol 10, No 1 January 2021

条目9a、8d

emboli and a large left pleural effusion. Despite appropriate treatment with therapeutic anticoagulation, placement of an indwelling pleural catheter, and continuation of alectinib, the patient developed worsening hypoxia on hospital day 11, requiring 8 L/min of oxygen by high-flow nasal cannula. A repeat CT scan of the chest at this time showed regression of the known pulmonary emboli and pleural effusion but interval development of diffuse ground-glass opacities and septal thickening (*Figure 1B*).

条目8b

Although sputum was positive for *Enterobacter cloacae*, the patient had no fever or leukocytosis and did not improve with piperacillin-tazobactam. Pulmonary edema was similarly considered to be unlikely given negative troponin levels (<0.055) and a recent echocardiogram showing normal left ventricular function without valvular abnormalities. Because the patient's precarious respiratory status prohibited bronchoscopy, methylprednisolone 60 mg intravenously (IV) daily was started empirically for grade 3 pneumonitis. By 48 hours later, his clinical status had improved significantly, with supplemental oxygen weaned to 4 L/min. Alectinib was discontinued at this time, and the patient continued to remain stable with decreasing oxygen requirements while he awaited eventual discharge to a skilled nursing facility.

条目9a、9b、8d、9c

条目9c、8d①

Approximately four weeks after hospitalization, while remaining on a slow steroid taper, a repeat CT scan of the chest, abdomen, and pelvis showed resolving ground-glass opacities (*Figure 1C*). However, there was also evidence of tumor growth, and therefore, following a careful discussion of the potential risks and alternatives, he started second-line lorlatinib 100 mg daily a few weeks later. After 10 weeks on lorlatinib, repeat CT scan of the chest, abdomen, and pelvis showed only faint residual ground-glass opacities, and the patient was asymptomatic without hypoxia despite having been weaned to prednisone 2 mg daily, indicating no recurrence of pneumonitis (*Figure 1D*). Unfortunately, the CT scan also revealed progression in the lung and left adrenal gland, and a MRI of the brain showed new lesions in the left temporal horn and left frontal lobe. Lorlatinib was discontinued due to lack of efficacy, and the patient was transitioned to hospice care. He passed away shortly thereafter, with overall survival (OS) lasting approximately 7 months from the time of diagnosis.

条目9c、8d②

条目8d、9c

条目10b

Case #2

A 66 years old Caucasian, never-smoking woman with a history of depression presented in 2018 with several weeks of intermittent pain in the right upper back. A CT scan of the chest, abdomen, and pelvis showed a 2.9 cm × 2.6 cm spiculated lesion in the right inferior hilar region of the lung without diffuse parenchymal disease (*Figure 2A*). Additional findings included subcarinal and hilar lymphadenopathy, multiple liver lesions measuring up to 2.5 cm, and a nodular density near the left adrenal gland. Biopsy of a single liver lesion revealed a CK7+, TTF1+ lung adenocarcinoma with high PD-L1 expression (>50%). As a result of the patient's symptom burden and the inadequate tissue available for next-generation sequencing (NGS), she was started on pembrolizumab 200 mg IV every 3 weeks for stage IV (cT1cN2M1c) NSCLC. After two cycles of immunotherapy, her disease was found to have progressed, and therefore, she was switched to second-line alectinib 600 mg twice daily based on repeat molecular sequencing that revealed an *EML4-ALK* rearrangement.

On day 26 of alectinib, the patient presented to the hospital with acute dyspnea and hypoxia requiring 100% FiO2 by face mask. A CT scan of the chest showed new diffuse, bilateral ground-glass opacities along with moderate, bilateral pleural effusions (*Figure 2B*). A basic infectious work-up, consisting of blood and sputum cultures, was unrevealing. The patient was offered bronchoscopy for further diagnostic evaluation but declined. Therefore, given clinical suspicion for grade 3 pneumonitis secondary to alectinib, her cancer therapy was empirically discontinued, and she was started on methylprednisolone 40 mg IV every 8 hours in addition to broad-spectrum antibiotics. Within 48 hours, the patient's condition rapidly improved, and by hospital day 5, she was weaned off all supplemental oxygen and safely discharged from the hospital.

Three weeks following hospitalization, while remaining on a slow steroid taper, a repeat CT scan of the chest showed complete radiographic resolution of ground-glass opacities (*Figure 2C*). The patient therefore began third-line carboplatin, area under the curve (AUC) (5), plus pemetrexed 500 mg/m^2 but she developed further tumor progression after two cycles. Following a detailed discussion of the risks and benefits, she was switched to fourth-line lorlatinib 75 mg daily while also remaining on dexamethasone 1 mg twice daily for chronic back pain. An interval PET-CT scan subsequently demonstrated a near complete response with resolution of lesions in the right middle lung and liver. The patient has thus far remained on lorlatinib for >10 months without clinical or radiographic evidence of recurrent DI-ILD (*Figure 2D*).

Both patients provided informed consent for the

Transl Lung Cancer Res 2021;10(1):487-495 | http://dx.doi.org/10.21037/tlcr-20-564

患者在住院第11天出现了严重缺氧，给予高流量鼻导管吸氧（8 L/min）。胸部CT显示肺栓塞和胸腔积液已经消退，但出现了弥漫性磨玻璃样不透明物和房间隔增厚。患者痰液中的梭状芽孢杆菌呈阳性，但患者未发热，使用哌拉西林−他唑巴坦也没有改善。

条目8b：诊断评估　诊断方面的挑战，如是否有条件开展检查、费用或文化挑战

报告到位。肌钙蛋白水平阴性，且超声心动图显示左心室功能正常，无瓣膜异常，因此排除肺水肿。由于患者呼吸状况不稳定，无法进行支气管镜检查。

条目9a：治疗干预 治疗干预的类型，如药物、手术、预防、自我护理等
条目9b：治疗干预 治疗干预的管理，如剂量、强度、持续时间
条目8d：诊断评估 预后，如肿瘤学中的分期（如适用）
条目9c：治疗干预 治疗干预的变化，需要提供改变理由

报告到位。静脉注射甲强龙60 mg，48 h后，病情得到改善，氧流量改为4 L/min。停用艾乐替尼后，患者病情稳定。

条目9c：治疗干预 治疗干预的变化，需要提供改变理由
条目8d①：诊断评估 预后，如肿瘤学中的分期（如适用）

报告到位。住院后约4周，在保持甲强龙缓慢减量的同时，CT扫描显示磨玻璃状的不透明物正在消失。然而，肿瘤也在生长。

条目9c：治疗干预 治疗干预的变化，需要提供改变理由
条目8d②：诊断评估 预后，如肿瘤学中的分期（如适用）

报告到位。更改方案，开始服用二线抗肿瘤药物劳拉替尼（100 mg/d）。10周后，CT扫描显示只有微弱的残留磨玻璃不透明物，且停用甲强龙后患者没有缺氧症状，肺炎没有复发。

条目8d：诊断评估 预后，如肿瘤学中的分期（如适用）
条目9c：治疗干预 治疗干预的变化，需要提供改变理由

报告到位。同时，CT扫描也显示肺部和左肾上腺都有进展，头部MRI显示左颞角和左额叶有新病变，因此停用劳拉替尼。

条目10b：随访和结局 重要的后续诊断和其他测试结果

报告到位。患者被转入临终关怀，作者一直保持了对患者的随访，患者不久后去世，总生存期约为7个月。

Translational Lung Cancer Research, Vol 10, No 1 January 2021

emboli and a large left pleural effusion. Despite appropriate treatment with therapeutic anticoagulation, placement of an indwelling pleural catheter, and continuation of alectinib, the patient developed worsening hypoxia on hospital day 11, requiring 8 L/min of oxygen by high-flow nasal cannula. A repeat CT scan of the chest at this time showed regression of the known pulmonary emboli and pleural effusion but interval development of diffuse ground-glass opacities and septal thickening (*Figure 1B*). Although sputum was positive for *Enterobacter cloacae*, the patient had no fever or leukocytosis and did not improve with piperacillin-tazobactam. Pulmonary edema was similarly considered to be unlikely given negative troponin levels (<0.055) and a recent echocardiogram showing normal left ventricular function without valvular abnormalities. Because the patient's precarious respiratory status prohibited bronchoscopy, methylprednisolone 60 mg intravenously (IV) daily was started empirically for grade 3 pneumonitis. By 48 hours later, his clinical status had improved significantly, with supplemental oxygen weaned to 4 L/min. Alectinib was discontinued at this time, and the patient continued to remain stable with decreasing oxygen requirements while he awaited eventual discharge to a skilled nursing facility.

Approximately four weeks after hospitalization, while remaining on a slow steroid taper, a repeat CT scan of the chest, abdomen, and pelvis showed resolving ground-glass opacities (*Figure 1C*). However, there was also evidence of tumor growth, and therefore, following a careful discussion of the potential risks and alternatives, he started second-line lorlatinib 100 mg daily a few weeks later. After 10 weeks on lorlatinib, repeat CT scan of the chest, abdomen, and pelvis showed only faint residual ground-glass opacities, and the patient was asymptomatic without hypoxia despite having been weaned to prednisone 2 mg daily, indicating no recurrence of pneumonitis (*Figure 1D*). Unfortunately, the CT scan also revealed progression in both the lung and left adrenal gland, and a MRI of the brain showed new lesions in the left temporal horn and left frontal lobe. Lorlatinib was discontinued due to lack of efficacy, and the patient was transitioned to hospice care. He passed away shortly thereafter, with overall survival (OS) lasting approximately 7 months from the time of diagnosis.

条目 5a、5c

Case #2

A 66 years old Caucasian, never-smoking woman with a history of depression presented in 2018 with several

weeks of intermittent pain in the right upper back. A CT scan of the chest, abdomen, and pelvis showed a 2.9 cm × 2.6 cm spiculated lesion in the right inferior hilar region of the lung without diffuse parenchymal disease (*Figure 2A*). Additional findings included subcarinal and hilar lymphadenopathy, multiple liver lesions measuring up to 2.5 cm, and a nodular density near the left adrenal gland. Biopsy of a single liver lesion revealed a CK7+, TTF1+ lung adenocarcinoma with high PD-L1 expression (>50%).

条目6

As a result of the patient's symptom burden and the inadequate tissue available for next-generation sequencing (NGS), she was started on pembrolizumab 200 mg IV every 3 weeks for stage IV (cT1cN2M1c) NSCLC. After two cycles of immunotherapy, her disease was found to have progressed, and therefore, she was switched to second-line alectinib 600 mg twice daily based on repeat molecular sequencing that revealed an *EML4-ALK* rearrangement.

条目9a、8d、9c

条目5b

On day 26 of alectinib, the patient presented to the hospital with acute dyspnea and hypoxia requiring 100% FiO2 by face mask. A CT scan of the chest showed new diffuse, bilateral ground-glass opacities along with moderate, bilateral pleural effusions (*Figure 2B*). A basic infectious work-up, consisting of blood and sputum cultures, was unrevealing. The patient was offered bronchoscopy for further diagnostic evaluation but declined. Therefore, given clinical suspicion for grade 3 pneumonitis secondary to alectinib, her cancer therapy was empirically discontinued, and she was started on methylprednisolone 40 mg IV every 8 hours in addition to broad-spectrum antibiotics. Within 48 hours, the patient's condition rapidly improved, and by hospital day 5, she was weaned off all supplemental oxygen and safely discharged from the hospital.

条目6、8a、8b

条目8c、9c

条目8d

Three weeks following hospitalization, while remaining on a slow steroid taper, a repeat CT scan of the chest showed complete radiographic resolution of ground-glass opacities (*Figure 2C*). The patient therefore began third-line carboplatin, area under the curve (AUC) (5), plus pemetrexed 500 mg/m² but she developed further tumor progression after two cycles. Following a detailed discussion of the risks and benefits, she was switched to fourth-line lorlatinib 75 mg daily while also remaining on dexamethasone 1 mg twice daily for chronic back pain. An interval PET-CT scan subsequently demonstrated a near complete response with resolution of lesions in the right middle lung and liver. The patient has thus far remained on lorlatinib for >10 months without clinical or radiographic evidence of recurrent DI-ILD (*Figure 2D*).

条目9c、8d

条目9c、8d

Both patients provided informed consent for the

条目10b

Transl Lung Cancer Res 2021;10(1):487-495 | http://dx.doi.org/10.21037/tlcr-20-564

第二个病例

条目5a：患者信息　去除患者身份的具体信息
条目5c：患者信息　医疗、家庭和社会心理史，包括相关的遗传信息

报告到位。报告了患者种族、年龄、性别、吸烟史与疾病相关的信息；患者有社会心理病史，2018年出现右上背间歇性疼痛数周。

条目6：临床发现　描述重要的检查和重要的临床发现

报告到位。详细描述了各种检查结果及临床发现，胸部、腹部和骨盆的CT扫描显示有肿瘤，右下肺区棘状病变。其他检查发现隆突下和肺门淋巴结肿大，多发肝脏病变，左侧肾上腺附近有密度结节。肝脏活检显示CK7⁺，TTF1⁺肺腺癌，PD-L1高表达。

条目9a：治疗干预　治疗干预的类型，如药物、手术、预防、自我护理等
条目8d：诊断评估　预后，如肿瘤学中的分期（如适用）
条目9c：治疗干预　治疗干预的变化，需要提供改变理由

报告到位。患者开始接受派姆单抗200 mg静脉注射，每3周1次（这里的叙述比较详细，建议参考）。经过2个周期的免疫治疗后，疾病进展，根据重复的分子测序发现EML4–ALK重排，改为二线抗肿瘤药物艾乐替尼600 mg，每天2次。

条目5b：患者信息　主诉和症状

报告到位。在使用艾乐替尼的第26天，由于急性呼吸困难和缺氧，患者到医院就诊。

条目6：临床发现　描述重要的检查和重要的临床发现
条目8a：诊断评估　诊断检查，如体格检查、实验室检查、影像学检查、调查
条目8b：诊断评估　诊断方面的挑战，如是否有条件开展检查、费用或文化挑战

报告到位。胸部CT扫描显示新的弥漫性双侧磨玻璃样不透明物，以及中度的双侧胸腔积液。基本的感染性检查，包括血液和痰液培养，都没有发现问题。为进一步诊断评估，需要进行支气管镜检查，但患者拒绝。

条目8c：诊断评估　诊断，包括鉴别诊断
条目9c：治疗干预　治疗干预的变化，需要提供改变理由

报告到位。怀疑是继发于艾乐替尼的3级肺炎，化疗被中止，并开始使用甲强龙40 mg，每8小时1次，加用广谱抗生素。

条目8d：诊断评估　预后，如肿瘤学中的分期（如适用）

报告到位。经上述处理后，患者的病情迅速好转，到了第5天，无需吸氧，患者出院。

条目9c：治疗干预　治疗干预的变化，需要提供改变理由
条目8d：诊断评估　预后，如肿瘤学中的分期（如适用）

报告到位。住院3周后，在保持甲强龙缓慢减量的同时，胸部CT扫描显示磨玻璃样斑点完全消失。患者改用三线抗肿瘤药物卡铂联合培美曲塞（500 mg/m²），但2个周期后肿瘤出现进展。

条目9c：治疗干预　治疗干预的变化，需要提供改变理由

条目8d：诊断评估　预后，如肿瘤学中的分期（如适用）

报告到位。改为四线抗肿瘤药物劳拉替尼，75 mg/d，同时还因慢性背痛而继续服用地塞米松1 mg，每天2次。随后PET–CT扫描显示，右中肺和肝脏病变得到控制，几乎完全缓解。

条目10b：随访和结果　重要的后续诊断和其他测试结果

报告到位。截至撰稿时间点，该患者已经服用劳拉替尼超过10个月，没有复发DI–ILD。

条目7

490　　　　　　　　　　　　　　　　　Myall et al. Case series of lorlatinib following alectinib-induced pneumonitis

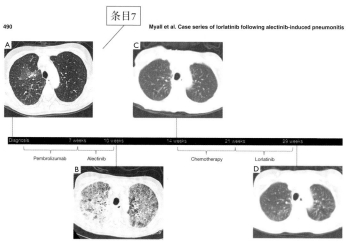

Figure 2 Serial CT images of the chest were collected in the second patient from the time of diagnosis through follow-up on lorlatinib. At the time of diagnosis with NSCLC, no parenchymal abnormalities were observed aside from the primary tumor (not shown) (A). When the patient was hospitalized with hypoxia and respiratory symptoms on day 26 of alectinib, diffuse ground-glass opacities involving the entirety of both lung fields were now noted (B). Approximately 3 weeks after discharge from the hospital, while the patient remained on corticosteroids and off alectinib, the previously seen parenchymal abnormalities were resolved (C). Despite later switching to lorlatinib, the lungs remained clear without recurrent ground-glass opacities (D).

条目13

reporting of their relevant medical histories in this manuscript. All procedures performed in studies involving human participants were in accordance with the ethical standards of the institutional and/or national research committee(s) and with the Helsinki Declaration (as revised in 2013).

Discussion

To our knowledge, the safety of lorlatinib in patients with a history of DI-ILD has not been previously reported. Although the incidence of DI-ILD secondary to ALK targeted therapy is low, it carries a 50% risk of mortality according to one prior case series (6). The occurrence of this serious adverse event also has the potential to impact long-term cancer control by limiting further use of highly effective ALK inhibitors. For these reasons, it is important

not only to understand the management of DI-ILD in the acute setting but also to recognize what constitutes safe, effective anti-cancer therapy following recovery from DI-ILD.

Drug-induced ILD is characterized by progressive respiratory symptoms and radiographic pulmonary abnormalities following exposure to a culprit medication (7). In the case of ALK inhibitors, in particular, DI-ILD has been reported in small numbers of patients across multiple prospective trials (8-11). A pooled analysis of four studies investigating crizotinib (PROFILE 1001/1005/1007/1014), for example, reported *de novo* DI-ILD in 1.2% of patients (6). Like cases of DI-ILD occurring secondary to other medications, common symptoms include fever, dyspnea, and cough, often beginning within 1–2 months of drug initiation (6). Although alectinib has now replaced crizotinib as first-line therapy in patients with

 Transl Lung Cancer Res 2021;10(1):487-495 | http://dx.doi.org/10.21037/tlcr-20-564

条目11b

条目7：时间轴　以时间轴的形式组织诊治照护信息，包括历史信息和当前信息

和第一个病例类似，作者详细按时间轴报告了治疗经过和对应的影像学改变。同样地，除了注明化疗药以外，还需要补充何时开始使用甲强龙、何时减量，同时建议作者补充患者的随访结果。除了第几周这样的表述外，最好明确给出年月。

条目13：知情同意　患者是否知情同意？如有需要，请提供知情同意书

报告到位。作者说明两位患者都提供了知情同意书。

条目11c

条目11b

491

metastatic, *ALK*-rearranged NSCLC, its risk of causing DI-ILD appears to be similar. In the J-ALEX trial, for example, DI-ILD occurred in 8% of Japanese patients in both the alectinib and crizotinib arms (12). While drug discontinuation secondary to DI-ILD was less common with alectinib than crizotinib (0.7% *vs.* 3.3%) in the international ALEX trial, the small number of patients developing DI-ILD in either arm limited statistical comparison (1). Conversely, a meta-analysis of 18 studies found that the lower incidence of all-grade DI-ILD in patients receiving alectinib versus crizotinib (1.62% *vs.* 2.68%) did not reach statistical significance (P=0.092) (13).

As a clinical entity, DI-ILD encompasses a number of distinct histologic patterns in the lung including diffuse alveolar damage, organizing pneumonia, and eosinophilic pneumonia, among others (7,14). Diffuse alveolar damage, in particular, is defined pathologically by hyaline membrane formation and exudative edema, and it often manifests clinically with hypoxia and bilateral ground-glass opacities suggestive of adult respiratory distress syndrome (ARDS) (14,15). In the case of DI-ILD secondary to ALK inhibitors, it has been suggested that diffuse alveolar damage correlates with an acute and severely symptomatic form of the disease in which patients are at risk for decompensation and death without discontinuation of ALK targeted therapy (16). On the other hand, a delayed form of DI-ILD occurring several months after the start of ALK targeted therapy is characterized by fewer symptoms and focal, less prominent ground-glass opacities (16). Although pathologic data was not obtained in our two patients, their clinical presentation was similar to that of prior cases of DI-ILD that have been associated with diffuse alveolar damage on post-mortem evaluation (17,18).

Because of the mortality associated with DI-ILD, the question of whether or not to restart ALK targeted therapy in patients who have a history of DI-ILD requires careful consideration. A limited number of previous case reports have described the successful use of crizotinib, ceritinib, alectinib, or brigatinib in patients with *ALK*-rearranged NSCLC who have recovered from DI-ILD secondary to ALK targeted therapy (*Table 1*) (19-31). In some of these cases, however, patients resumed ALK targeted therapy after having mild and/or delayed presentations of DI-ILD marked by focal opacities (19,20,26,28). As discussed above, this may represent a distinct form of DI-ILD for which continuation of ALK inhibitor therapy is not prohibited (16). In comparison, both patients in our series presented with acute, severe DI-ILD, and thus, their subsequent tolerance

of lorlatinib was notable. While it is unclear to what extent the ongoing use of steroids played a protective role in our patients, the doses being used at the time of starting lorlatinib were much lower than the treatment doses typically indicated for active DI-ILD.

Although DI-ILD is uncommon, potential risk factors for the disease have been previously identified in patients receiving ALK targeted therapy. These include older age, Japanese ethnicity, positive smoking history, and the presence of concurrent pleural effusions (6,32). A more recently identified risk factor that may have played a role in the development of DI-ILD in our second patient, in particular, is the use of immune checkpoint inhibitor therapy prior to TKI therapy. In multiple series of patients with *epidermal growth factor receptor* (*EGFR*)-mutated NSCLC, for example, the incidence of pneumonitis has been found to be higher in those patients who have received PD-1/PD-L1 inhibitors prior to EGFR targeted therapy (33,34). A similar phenomenon has been demonstrated in patients with *ALK*-rearranged NSCLC in whom the incidence of grade 3–4 transaminitis has been shown to be significantly higher in patients receiving checkpoint inhibitors prior to crizotinib [45.5% versus 8.1% for elevated alanine transaminase (ALT) and 36.4% versus 3.4% for elevated aspartate transaminase (AST)] (35).

Together, these results suggest that the sequential use of checkpoint inhibitors before TKI therapy may exacerbate the risk of immune-related and/or TKI-related adverse events such as DI-ILD. For those patients with severely symptomatic disease at the time of diagnosis, starting therapy immediately may be necessary prior to knowing the results of *EGFR* and/or *ALK* molecular testing. However, this is challenging in patients who ultimately have *ALK*-rearranged NSCLC given that *ALK* rearrangements have been associated with PD-L1 expression but are not predictive of response to immunotherapy (36,37). Therefore, given both the lack of efficacy and the increased risk of side-effects, checkpoint inhibitors should be deferred while awaiting molecular results in patients who, by virtue of their age or non-smoking status, have a high pretest probability of testing positive for a targetable driver mutation. Furthermore, studies suggest that patients are at greatest risk for adverse events when TKI therapy is initiated within 3 months of discontinuing checkpoint inhibition (34). However, pharmacodynamic studies also suggest that immune checkpoint inhibitors may have a continued effect on T-cells long after administration (38).

Transl Lung Cancer Res 2021;10(1):487-495 | http://dx.doi.org/10.21037/tlcr-20-564

61

病例系列的讨论

条目11b：讨论 引用参考文献以展开对相关医学文献的讨论

报告到位。作者首先强调了DI-ILD的高病死率，以及可能通过限制ALK抑制药的使用而影响癌症控制，因此应对DI-ILD管理引起重视。其次，分析了几篇关于使用艾乐替尼与克唑替尼是否导致DI-ILD的研究，仍未得出一致的结论。再次，作者探讨出现DI-ILD后是否应暂停ALK抑制药，结果仍存在争议。最后，用表格总结了在DI-ILD后使用ALK抑制药并恢复的非小细胞肺癌患者的案例报告，进一步支持了DI-ILD后ALK抑制药的使用。在该病例系列中，两名患者都在使用艾乐替尼后出现了严重的DI-ILD，在换用劳拉替尼后未再出现且有较好的耐药性。

条目11c：讨论 给出结论的科学依据，包括对可能原因的评估

报告到位。DI-ILD潜在危险因素有年龄、种族、吸烟史等，同时还包括在

Table 1 Prior case reports describing ALK inhibitor use after drug-induced pneumonitis

Case Report	Demographics	Initial ALK TKI	Time to Onset of DI-ILD[1]	Re-treatment ALK TKI
Asai et al. (19)	70 yo F	Crizotinib	35 days	Crizotinib
Asai et al. (20)	60 yo M	Crizotinib	50 days	Crizotinib
Bender et al. (21)	53 yo F	Ceritinib	7 months	Crizotinib Brigatinib
Chino et al. (22)	46 yo F	Crizotinib	47 days	Alectinib
Doménech et al. (23)	45 yo F	Crizotinib	9 days	Brigatinib
Fujiuchi et al. (24)	70 yo F	Crizotinib	60 days	Alectinib
Hwang et al. (25)	46 yo F	Alectinib	28 days	Alectinib
Lim et al. (26)	45 yo F	Ceritinib	6 months	Ceritinib
Maka et al. (27)	47 yo F	Crizotinib	60 days	Crizotinib
Nitawaki et al. (28)[2]	57 yo M	Alectinib	33 days	Alectinib
	64 yo F	Alectinib	12 months	Alectinib
Nukaga et al. (29)	63 yo M	Crizotinib	27 days	Alectinib
Tachihara et al. (30)	70 yo M	Crizotinib	25 days	Crizotinib
Yanagisawa et al. (31)	53 yo F	Crizotinib	10 days	Crizotinib

[1]Time of onset is defined is the duration in days or months from initiation of ALK targeted therapy to presentation with DI-ILD; [2]Two cases described in the same case series. ALK, anaplastic lymphoma kinase; TKI, tyrosine kinase inhibitor; DI-ILD, drug-induced interstitial lung disease.

Therefore, it was notable that the second patient in this series tolerated lorlatinib despite both her history of severe DI-ILD and recent exposure to immunotherapy just a few months prior.

Drug-induced ILD often remains a diagnosis of exclusion, although pathologic evaluation can provide supporting data (7,14,15). Bronchoscopic evaluation or biopsy was prohibited in both patients in this series, either by patient choice or clinical instability. Nonetheless, the acute onset of radiographic abnormalities and rapid clinical recovery with steroids and discontinuation of alectinib strengthened the diagnosis of DI-ILD in both cases and encourages the reporting of larger patient cohorts in the future to confirm the hypotheses developed here. Another potential limitation of this case series is the lack of long-term follow-up data for the first patient who showed evidence of progression of NSCLC on first surveillance imaging after starting lorlatinib. While many severe cases of DI-ILD occur acutely, reports of long-term safety data will be important in the future to assess the potential for delayed adverse events secondary to lorlatinib.

In summary, we present two patients who tolerated lorlatinib without recurrent symptoms after developing severe, acute DI-ILD on alectinib. Although confirmation is warranted in additional patients, these results offer initial safety data suggesting that lorlatinib may be a reasonable alternative therapy to consider in patients who have recovered from DI-ILD. Given the efficacy of ALK inhibitors in patients with *ALK*-rearranged NSCLC, this offers hope that patients may continue to tolerate and benefit from ALK inhibitor therapy even after the development of significant grade ≥3 DI-ILD.

Acknowledgments

The authors would like to thank the patients who are described in this manuscript. We would also like to thank the medical staff members who have provided care for the patients both in the hospital and the outpatient setting.
Funding: None.

Footnote

Reporting Checklist: The authors have completed the CARE reporting checklist. Available at http://dx.doi.org/10.21037/tlcr-20-564

          Transl Lung Cancer Res 2021;10(1):487-495 | http://dx.doi.org/10.21037/tlcr-20-564

TKI治疗之前使用免疫抑制药治疗。因此，鉴于缺乏疗效和增加的不良反应风险，对于那些因年龄或不吸烟而具有较高的可靶向驱动基因突变预检阳性概率的患者，应推迟使用免疫抑制药，以等待分子检查结果（EGFR、ALK等）。

条目11a：讨论 对本病例报告的优点和局限性进行科学讨论

报告到位。没有回避问题。两名患者都拒绝行支气管镜评估或活检；缺乏第一个患者的长期随访数据。

条目11d：讨论 用一个无参考文献的段落来给出结论，说明本病例报告的主要启示

报告到位。可以为临床实践提供指导：对于已从DI-ILD中恢复的患者，劳拉替尼可能是一种安全的治疗选择，为出现≥3级DI-ILD后仍能继续耐受ALK抑制药的患者提供了治疗希望。

Translational Lung Cancer Research, Vol 10, No 1 January 2021 493

Peer Review File: Available at http://dx.doi.org/10.21037/tlcr-20-564

Conflicts of Interest: All authors have completed the ICMJE uniform disclosure form (available at http://dx.doi.org/10.21037/tlcr-20-564). Dr. Wakelee serves as an unpaid editorial board member of Translational Lung Cancer Research. Dr. Wakelee reports grants from Gilead; personal fees and non-financial support from AztraZeneca; personal fees and other from Xcovery, personal fees from Janssen, Daiichi Sankyo, INC, Helsinn, and Mirati; non-financial support from Takeda, and CellWorks; non-financial support and other from Genentech/Roche, Merck; non-financial support from Clinical Care Options Oncology, LLC, Fishawack Facilitate LTD, Medscape, Onclive/Intellisphere LLC, Phillips Gilmore Oncology (2018), Physicians Education Resource LLC/MJH (Targeted Oncology), Potomac Center for Medical Education (Rockpointe), Prime Oncology LLC (2018), Primo (2018), Research to Practice; personal fees from UpToDate; non-financial support from WebMD Health, Novartis, RGCON - Rajiv Gandi Conference, JLCS - Japanese Lung Cancer Society, KSMO - Korean Society of Medical Oncology, Stanford University, ITMIG, other from ACEA Biosciences; other from Arrys Therapeutics, AztraZeneca/MedImmune, BMS, Celgene, Clovis Oncology, Exelixis, Lilly, Pfizer, Pharmacyclics; which are all outside the submitted work. The other authors have no conflicts of interest to declare.

Ethical Statement: The authors are accountable for all aspects of the work in ensuring that questions related to the accuracy or integrity of any part of the work are appropriately investigated and resolved. Both patients provided informed consent for the reporting of their relevant medical histories in this manuscript. All procedures performed in studies involving human participants were in accordance with the ethical standards of the institutional and/or national research committee(s) and with the Helsinki Declaration (as revised in 2013).

Open Access Statement: This is an Open Access article distributed in accordance with the Creative Commons Attribution-NonCommercial-NoDerivs 4.0 International License (CC BY-NC-ND 4.0), which permits the non-commercial replication and distribution of the article with the strict proviso that no changes or edits are made and the original work is properly cited (including links to both the formal publication through the relevant DOI and the license). See: https://creativecommons.org/licenses/by-nc-nd/4.0/.

References

1. Camidge DR, Dziadziuszko R, Peters S, et al. Updated Efficacy and Safety Data and Impact of the EML4-ALK Fusion Variant on the Efficacy of Alectinib in Untreated ALK-Positive Advanced Non-Small Cell Lung Cancer in the Global Phase III ALEX Study. J Thorac Oncol 2019;14:1233-43.
2. Shaw AT, Felip E, Bauer TM, et al. Lorlatinib in non-small-cell lung cancer with ALK or ROS1 rearrangement: an international, multicentre, open-label, single-arm first-in-man phase 1 trial. Lancet Oncol 2017;18:1590-9.
3. Solomon BJ, Besse B, Bauer TM, et al. Lorlatinib in patients with ALK-positive non-small-cell lung cancer: results from a global phase 2 study. Lancet Oncol 2018;19:1654-67.
4. Shaw AT, Solomon BJ, Besse B, et al. ALK Resistance Mutations and Efficacy of Lorlatinib in Advanced Anaplastic Lymphoma Kinase-Positive Non-Small-Cell Lung Cancer. J Clin Oncol 2019;37:1370-9.
5. Gagnier JJ, Kienle G, Altman DG, et al. The CARE guidelines: consensus-based clinical case reporting guideline development. J Med Case Rep 2013;7:223.
6. Yoneda KY, Scranton JR, Cadogan MA, et al. Interstitial Lung Disease Associated With Crizotinib in Patients With Advanced Non-Small-Cell Lung Cancer: Independent Review of Four PROFILE Trials. Clin Lung Cancer 2017;18:472-9.
7. Camus P, Fanton A, Bonniaud P, et al. Interstitial lung disease induced by drugs and radiation. Respiration 2004;71:301-26.
8. Peters S, Camidge DR, Shaw AT, et al. Alectinib versus Crizotinib in Untreated ALK-Positive Non-Small-Cell Lung Cancer. N Engl J Med 2017;377:829-38.
9. Camidge DR, Kim HR, Ahn MJ, et al. Brigatinib versus Crizotinib in ALK-Positive Non-Small-Cell Lung Cancer. N Engl J Med 2018;379:2027-39.
10. Soria JC, Yan DSW, Chiari R, et al. First-line ceritinib versus platinum-based chemotherapy in advanced ALK-rearranged non-small-cell lung cancer (ASCEND-4): a randomised, open-label, phase 3 study. Lancet 2017;389:917-29.
11. Solomon BJ, Mok T, Kim DW, et al. First-line crizotinib versus chemotherapy in ALK-positive lung cancer. N Engl J Med 2014;371:2167-77.

12. Hida T, Nokihara H, Kondo M, et al. Alectinib versus crizotinib in patients with ALK-positive non-small-cell lung cancer (J-ALEX): an open-label, randomised phase 3 trial. Lancet 2017;390:29-39.

13. Suh CH, Kim KW, Pyo J, et al. The incidence of ALK inhibitor-related pneumonitis in advanced non-small-cell lung cancer patients: A systematic review and meta-analysis. Lung Cancer 2019;132:79-86.

14. Müller NL, White DA, Jiang H, et al. Diagnosis and management of drug-associated interstitial lung disease. Br J Cancer 2004;91:S24-S30.

15. Min JH, Lee HY, Lim H, et al. Drug-induced interstitial lung disease in tyrosine kinase inhibitor therapy for non-small cell lung cancer: a review on current insight. Cancer Chemother Pharmacol 2011;68:1099-109.

16. Créquit P, Wislez M, Feith JF, et al. Crizotinib Associated with Ground-Glass Opacity Predominant Pattern Interstitial Lung Disease: A Retrospective Observational Cohort Study with a Systematic Literature Review. J Thorac Oncol 2015;10:1148-55.

17. Ono A, Takahashi T, Oishi T, et al. Acute lung injury with alveolar hemorrhage as adverse drug reaction related to crizotinib. J Clin Oncol 2013;31:e417-9.

18. Tamiya A, Okamoto I, Miyazaki M, et al. Severe acute interstitial lung disease after crizotinib therapy in a patient with EML4-ALK-positive non-small-cell lung cancer. J Clin Oncol 2013;31:e15-7.

19. Asai N, Yamaguchi E, Kubo A. Successful crizotinib rechallenge after crizotinib-induced interstitial lung disease in patients with advanced non-small-cell lung cancer. Clin Lung Cancer 2014;15:e33-5.

20. Asai N, Yokoi T, Yamaguchi E, et al. Successful crizotinib rechallenge after crizotinib-induced organizing pneumonia in anaplastic lymphoma kinase-rearranged non-small cell lung cancer. Case Rep Oncol 2014;7:681-4.

21. Bender L, Meyer G, Quoix E, et al. Ceritinib-related interstitial lung disease improving after treatment cessation without recurrence under either crizotinib or brigatinib: a case report. Ann Transl Med 2019;7:106.

22. Chino H, Sekine A, Kitamura H, et al. Successful treatment with alectinib after crizotinib-induced interstitial lung disease. Lung Cancer 2015;90:610-3.

23. Doménech M, Jové M, Aso S, et al. Successful treatment with brigatinib in a patient with ALK-rearranged lung adenocarcinoma who developed crizotinib-induced interstitial lung disease. Lung Cancer 2018;119:99-102.

24. Fujiuchi S, Fujita Y, Ssaki T, et al. Successful alectinib treatment after crizotinib-induced interstitial lung disease.

Respirol Case Rep 2016;4:e00156.

25. Hwang A, Iskandar A, Dasanu C. Successful re-introduction of alectinib after inducing interstitial lung disease in a patient with lung cancer. J Oncol Pharm Pract 2019;25:1531-3.

26. Lim SM, An HJ, Park HS, et al. Organizing pneumonia resembling disease progression in a non-small-cell lung cancer patient receiving ceritinib: A case report. Medicine (Baltimore) 2018;97:e11646.

27. Maka VV, Krishnaswamy UM, Kumar AN, et al. Acute interstitial lung disease in a patient with anaplastic lymphoma kinase-positive non-small-cell lung cancer after crizotinib therapy. Oxf Med Case Reports 2014;2014:11-2.

28. Nitawaki T, Sakata Y, Kawamura K, et al. Case report: continued treatment with alectinib is possible for patients with lung adenocarcinoma with drug-induced interstitial lung disease. BMC Pulm Med 2017;17:173.

29. Nukaga S, Naoki K, Kamo T, et al. Alectinib as a treatment option following recovery from crizotinib-induced interstitial lung disease in patients with anaplastic lymphoma kinase-positive advanced non-small-cell lung cancer. Mol Clin Oncol 2016;4:1085-7.

30. Tachihara M, Kobayashi K, Ishikawa Y, et al. Successful crizotinib rechallenge after crizotinib-induced interstitial lung disease. Jpn J Clin Oncol 2014;44:762-4.

31. Yanagisawa S, Inoue A, Koarai A, et al. Successful crizotinib retreatment after crizotinib-induced interstitial lung disease. J Thorac Oncol 2013;8:e73-4.

32. Gemma A, Kusumoto M, Kurihara Y, et al. Interstitial Lung Disease Onset and Its Risk Factors in Japanese Patients With ALK-Positive NSCLC After Treatment With Crizotinib. J Thorac Oncol 2019;14:672-82.

33. Oshima Y, Tanimoto T, Yuji K, et al. EGFR-TKI-Associated Interstitial Pneumonitis in Nivolumab-Treated Patients With Non-Small Cell Lung Cancer. JAMA Oncol 2018;4:1112-5.

34. Schoenfeld AJ, Arbour KC, Rizvi H, et al. Severe immune-related adverse events are common with sequential PD-(L)1 blockade and osimertinib. Ann Oncol 2019;30:839-44.

35. Lin JJ, Chin E, Yeap BY, et al. Increased Hepatotoxicity Associated with Sequential Immune Checkpoint Inhibitor and Crizotinib Therapy in Patients with Non–Small Cell Lung Cancer. J Thorac Oncol 2019;14:135-40.

36. Ota K, Azuma K, Kawahara A, et al. Induction of PD-L1 Expression by the EML4-ALK Oncoprotein and Downstream Signaling Pathways in Non-Small Cell Lung Cancer. Clin Cancer Res 2015;21:4014-21.

Transl Lung Cancer Res 2021;10(1):487-495 | http://dx.doi.org/10.21037/tlcr-20-564

37. Gainor JF, Shaw AT, Sequist LV, et al. EGFR Mutations and ALK Rearrangements Are Associated with Low Response Rates to PD-1 Pathway Blockade in Non-Small Cell Lung Cancer: A Retrospective Analysis. Clin Cancer Res 2016;22:4585-93.

38. Brahmer JR, Drake CG, Wollner I, et al. Phase I study of single-agent anti-programmed death-1 (MDX-1106) in refractory solid tumors: safety, clinical, activity, pharmacodynamics, and immunologic correlates. J Clin Oncol 2010;28:3167-75.

Cite this article as: Myall NJ, Lei AQ, Wakelee HA. Safety of lorlatinib following alectinib-induced pneumonitis in two patients with *ALK*-rearranged non-small cell lung cancer: a case series. Transl Lung Cancer Res 2021;10(1):487-495. doi: 10.21037/tlcr-20-564

Transl Lung Cancer Res 2021;10(1):487-495 | http://dx.doi.org/10.21037/tlcr-20-564

作者：尚炳含，AME出版社
审核修订：张开平，AME出版社
校对：林瑶，AME出版社
　　　杨芳慧，AME出版社

AME Medical Journals

Founded in 2009, AME has been rapidly entering into the international market by embracing the highest editorial standards and cutting-edge publishing technologies. Till now, AME has published more than 60 peer-reviewed journals (13 indexed in Web of Science/SCIE, 7 indexed in Web of Science/ESCI and 20 indexed in PubMed), predominantly in English (some are translated into Chinese), covering various fields of medicine including oncology, pulmonology, cardiothoracic disease, andrology, urology and so forth (updated on Aug. 2022).

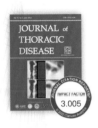 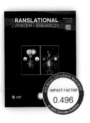 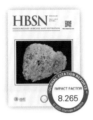 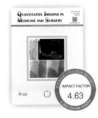 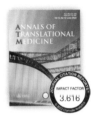

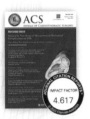 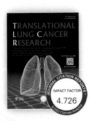 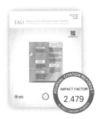 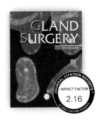 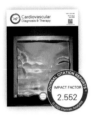

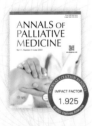 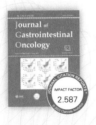 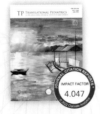 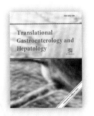 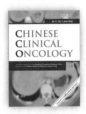

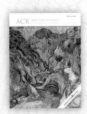 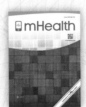 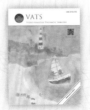 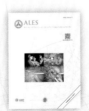 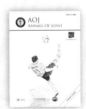

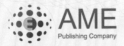
AME Publishing Company

Academic Made Easy, Excellent and Enthusiastic
破窗千里目、快乐搞学术

ISSN: 2523-1995

ACR AME CASE REPORTS

AN OPEN ACCESS EDUCATIONAL JOURNAL SHARING SIGNIFICANT CLINICAL CASES

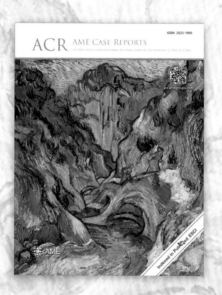

Features of *AME Case Report*

- Open access and peer-reviewed

- Indexed by PubMed/PMC and Emerging Sources Citation Index (ESCI)

- Publishing original and educationally valuable case reports in all medical disciplines

- A member of Committee on Publication Ethics (COPE)

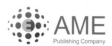

acr.amegroups.com

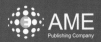
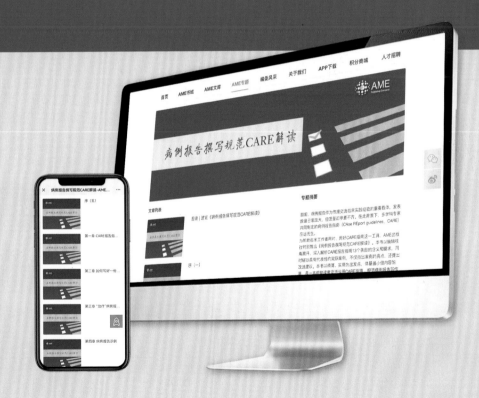